REVISIONING MEN'S LIVES

Revisioning
Men's
Lives

Gender, Intimacy, and Power

Terry A. Kupers

THE GUILFORD PRESS
New York   London

© The Guilford Press 1993
A Division of Guilford Publications, Inc.
72 Spring Street, New York, NY 10012

Printed in the United States of America

This book is printed on acid-free paper.

Last digit is print number: 9 8 7 6 5 4 3 2 1

Library of Congress Cataloging-in-Publication Data

Kupers, Terry Allen.
    Revisioning men's lives : gender, intimacy, and power / Terry A.
Kupers.
      p.   cm.
    Includes bibliographical references and index.
    ISBN 0-89862-993-4   0-89862-271-9 (pbk.)
    1. Men—Psychology.   2. Masculinity (Psychology)   3. Sex role.
I. Title
HQ1090.K86   1993
155.3'32—dc20   92-36142
                                                        CIP

Earlier versions of Chapters 1 and 2 appeared in *Tikkun*, July/August, 1990, and
March/April, 1991, respectively.

Acknowledgments

First, I want to thank my parents, Edward and Frances Kupers. Their loving collaboration in the parenting of six children has provided inspiration for me in my quest.

Since many of my ideas about gender have evolved in the consulting room, my clients deserve recognition and appreciation for their courage in taking risks and for all they have taught me.

The men's group I was part of in Los Angeles during the 1970s provided an indispensable forum for exploring the meaning of masculinity, as well as much needed support during a critical adult passage. Thanks, guys: Vic Aquilerra, Roger Bowers, Steve Kent, Mike Kogan, Cary Lowe, Bob Menard, Kevin O'Brien, and Stan Tropp.

Charles Bataille, Ram Gokul, Richard Lichtman, Gordon Murray, and Arlene Shmaeff read early drafts of this work and offered thoughtful comments and heartfelt encouragement.

Special thanks to all the other friends, family members and colleagues who have helped me along the tortuous path to writing this book. You know who you are.

Kitty Moore, my editor at the Guilford Press, provided invaluable support, sensitive feedback, and fine editing.

My three sons, Eric Kupers, Jake Ross, and Jesse Kupers, have provided inspiration and taught me quite a lot. The lessons are not always easy, sometimes we lose our way, but we always seem to find it again and the rewards are immense.

Arlene Shmaeff, my wife, has not only struggled with me on many of the issues discussed in these pages, but has also shared her ideas and stimulated me to think through the concepts.

Contents

Introduction

It's a Saturday, winter 1954. A basketball game is to be played in the park at 2. We arrive only to find the park closed for repairs. Jay says we can play at the schoolyard instead. Some of the boys ride bikes, others run. We get there several minutes later and find the gate locked. There is a six foot link fence with jagged edges at the top and no crossbar to hold onto while vaulting over. The ball is thrown over and several boys begin to climb the fence. I know I can climb to the top, but I am not certain I can make it over without tearing my jeans and cutting myself. I know several of the other boys will not be able to climb at all; they are too heavy or their feet are too big and they won't be able to squeeze their toes between the links. By now three or four boys are on the yard dribbling the ball, calling to the rest of us to climb over. Then comes the familiar taunt: "Don't be a girl!"

Among eleven-year-olds, gender lines are drawn sharply, cruelly. Potent men do certain things and only "chickens," "wimps," "losers," "weaklings," and "queers" do others. From childhood men are taught to toughen up, not to cry or be labeled a "sissy" or a "girl," not to "chicken out" of a fight or a dare, and to "go for it" in a game, a rivalry, or a project if we really want to win. And most important, we are supposed to really want to win. So we create our armor, the toughening and posturing, and the capacity to hide wounds, that we believe will guarantee no one will penetrate our defenses and get close enough to really do us harm. We can let down our guard with women, of course, and talk about our pain and our fear. Women are not a threat. Besides, who else can one talk with and take risks with? Many men are only able to feel fully alive when they are with a woman who adores them.

1

Our culture rewards men who are armored and posture well. One gains the satisfaction of being accepted in the ranks of the powerful, and, if lucky, one gains the admiration of those who worship power as well as the love of women who want to be with a winner—or so goes the American Dream. But there is a high price to pay. Men must be ever vigilant to avoid situations where betrayal is possible, and this means avoiding excessive intimacy with other men. Is it any wonder that, when things begin to go wrong—when men lose their jobs, their hopes, their partners, their hair, or their potency—they find themselves very much alone and in pain, unable to share with anyone their experience of inadequacy, feeling shame, and wondering if their problems might stem from a failure to be man enough.

At the basketball court we were rehearsing our parts in the traditional script: The boys with the real stuff would climb the fence and thereby win the right to shame the boys who could not climb over by calling them girls. I climbed the fence without tearing my pants and played. Three boys could not climb over. They turned to walk home. The boys in the yard did not have to jeer at them when they left, all the boys involved in the minidrama knew about humiliation. The trick was to act as if the feelings of the boys walking home did not matter. That was the part I found the most difficult. Not only had I been afraid to climb—the fact that I eventually scrambled over does not make the fear any more palatable to an eleven-year-old—but I also felt very bad for the boys who had to walk home. I felt ashamed about my part in ostracizing them, but could not talk about this with the other boys. At the time, I did not understand my shame; I was not yet aware one could act differently.

Boys regularly create bonds with each other by expressing a shared hatred toward women—a hatred that is, as we know, helpful to adolescent boys who are struggling desperately to develop a sense of self-esteem. My friends and I were learning to compete for a spot in the pecking order, and to mock males who were outdone. The next stage would be derisive talk of teenage males about the girls one had sex with in order to acquire status in the eyes of other boys. The pieces fall into place: competition among men, humiliation of the loser, objectification and devaluation of women, distrust and distancing between men, fear of weakness, stigmatization of homosexuality, and so forth.

Some adult men continue to obsess about competition, to humiliate underlings, to objectify and abuse women, to carefully avoid any sign of affection for and dependence on other men, to ignore their childrearing responsibilities, and to act out their feelings of inadequacy by harassing women and gays. In other words, they are still functioning as if the schoolyard rules were in force. These men are prone to feelings of inadequacy during hard times, and tend to intensify their domination over others when they feel inadequate. And these guys give men a bad name!

A man's merit, for good or ill, is traditionally based on his capacity to work and provide for a family. A large number of men are currently suffering from speedup, salary and benefit freezes, layoffs and unemployment, or merely the reality that it is harder to stretch a salary to cover expenses. Consider what might happen to a man who functions as if the schoolyard rules were in force when the factory where he has worked for many years closes because the company is moving to a Third World country where labor is cheaper and there are no unions or federal environmental regulations. Who does he blame? Certainly not the system, not the corporation that decided to close the plant and lay off the workers. With the decline in labor militancy over the last several decades, workers are less likely to join together to protest. Meanwhile, men have been trained—beginning with that familiar schoolyard scenario—to blame themselves, to feel inadequate as men. So this man, after he gets done kicking himself around the block a few times, might turn on his wife and children. He might get drunk, beat her, and leave the children with an indelible memory of domestic violence. In hard economic times, the incidence of alcoholism and domestic violence goes up very rapidly. Or the displacement of hostility toward women can be more subtle. For instance, many men stand by and watch as sexual harassment or gay-baiting goes on at work without saying anything, and explain that they would be quickly ostracized by "the guys" if they were to protest.

We need to be clear about the reasons some men misperceive their situation and blame women for their unfortunate plight. I believe it has to do with a precarious self-esteem system, and the assumption that women will prop men up so they won't fall over. Virginia Woolf (1929) said it very well: "Women have served all these centuries as looking-glasses possessing the magic and delicious power of reflecting the figure of man at twice its natural size" (p. 35). But in the process, of course, the woman is reduced to a fraction of her own size and power, because: "if women were not inferior, they would cease to enlarge."

To the extent men sustain their sense of power and virility at the expense of women, they begin to feel inadequate anew as women begin to stand up for themselves and refuse to be used as a mirror and shrunk in the process. So men blame women for their inadequacy, or intensify the attempt to control and use women. Thus, the man who is beaten down by the boss at work gets drunk, goes out and enlarges his string of sexual conquests, or comes home and beats his wife; as if to reassure himself he is still potent.

Not surprisingly, the incidences of sexual harassment at work, date rape, and male psychiatrists and psychotherapists engaging in sex with their female patients all seem to be rising. Perhaps it is a matter of us hearing more about the incidents because women are reporting them. I think it is a combination of higher incidences and more reporting. Think about the man's situation at work. It is more difficult, in an age of massive downscaling and layoffs, to climb up the hierarchy. But the economic downturn does not affect men's inner template, their view that their status in the hierarchy, their earning power, and their ability to provide for their families are the measures of their manliness. Men feel they are losing ground, and consequently feel inadequate. Meanwhile, they see women entering the workplace, they see minorities, they see gays coming out of the closet on account of affirmative action and laws that protect constitutional rights. So men blame women, minority members, and gays who seem to be doing better (the sad truth is, these groups are having an even harder time) and the incidence of sexual harassment, rape, gay-bashing, and other forms of discrimination, misogyny, and homophobia climb. At the same time, more men are lured by false cures for a faltering sense of manhood: workaholism, drugs and alcohol, conspicuous consumption, sexual conquests, pornography, and so forth.

Of course, this caricature does not describe all men. Far from it. A large number of men are repulsed by stereotypic male posturing, and the abuse of women, children, and gays. When the women's liberation movement blossomed in the late sixties and early seventies a large number of men who had serious reservations about the traditional script joined women in the struggle for gender equality. It seemed only fair. To fight for civil rights and peace felt right, but in that struggle men gave all the speeches while women were left with the burden of doing the housework, taking notes at meetings, and running off flyers on mimeograph machines. Something was wrong. When women began to protest that the division of labor was unfair, men of principle had to admit they were right. Some male activists did not support the principle of gender equality. But most did, and have continued to struggle for gender equality even if they are no longer as active in social struggles. Of course, that struggle threw into question the meaning of masculinity.

In the last twenty years, with heightened interest in male psychology and the emergence of a men's movement, a much larger number of men have begun to discover the links between traditional male armoring, the tendency for men to battle for dominance in hierarchies, men's feelings of inadequacy and shame, their isolation from each other, and the compensatory tendency to oppress women and gays. Today's men's movement is much larger than the group of men who came of age in the sixties and seventies. It includes members of ongoing men's groups, therapists and others who specialize in "working with men," anti-sexist and gay activists, men in recovery from drug and alcohol abuse, men who are avid readers of a growing men's literature, and those who attend men's meetings and gatherings.

But the men's movement is divided. Some men believe that merely by meeting together—in psychotherapy, in men's groups, or in men's gatherings and conferences—they can dramatically improve their situation. This group includes psychologists, men who lead and attend men's gatherings and subscribe to the "mythopoetic" school of thought, "men's rights" advocates, and a large group of men who are in recovery. Another group, the "political" or "pro-feminist" segment of the men's movement, believes it is the inequities inherent in our social relations that cause men's difficulties, and that straight men must join with women and gays in a struggle to radically transform those restrictive social relations. As I explain in Chapter Nine, I see no reason for the movement to remain divided; the men's movement can relate to the personal needs that cause men to seek change while remaining aware of the social tragedies that are unfolding in front of our eyes.

Then there is an even larger number of men who do not consider themselves part of any movement, but have transcended the traditional male role and can be tender and supportive toward the women in their lives, take seriously their role as fathers, and make it very clear, even to other guys, that they do not condone harassment and violence against women and gays. As a psychiatrist, I regularly hear from men in my consulting room what ails them. George is an example. He comes to my office complaining of depression and tells me he feels "inadequate as a man." His wife earns a higher salary than he does and he has been passed over for a promotion—he thinks it is because he refuses to stay at the office nights and come in weekends. I tell George I suspect that his wife is only able to be successful in her career because she knows he is home sharing childrearing responsibilities, and that his choice to go against the tide in this way requires a certain amount of courage. He seems to brighten and tells me that he could never be away from his family as much as someone in the fast track is expected to be.

What do men want? Men want to feel productive, successful, loved, virile and fully alive. The problem for men today is that we believe the only way to feel these things is to be powerful, and we define power in a very traditional, one-dimensional way as power over others. This is a trap! It is a trap for the man who affects the tough guy image, lording it over others but always living in fear of the inevitable moment of betrayal, defeat and humiliation. It is a trap for men like George who elect to share housekeeping and childrearing equally but then fear the derision of other men who might consider him a "wimp" or "Momma's boy" for doing so. And it is a trap for other men who do not fit either of these descriptions. Men are in great pain today, but their training for manhood makes it very difficult for them to identify the sources of the pain and reach out to others for help.

One man recently told me he has to follow orders on the job and he considers the superior who gives the orders to be less competent than he is, but because he is stuck in a lower place on the hierarchy than he feels he merits, he is unjustly forced to be submissive. Another man complains that his wife is not interested in sex, and this leaves him feeling undesired; this is why he regularly turns to pornography or goes to sexually oriented massage parlors. Men complain that they feel dead, empty inside, lack meaning in their lives, do not know why they should go on living. Or they say they feel depressed, impotent, anxious in the wake of a heart attack, or just plain uneasy. When I ask what they think is wrong, they do not know; or they tell me that their partner is the one who tells them they need therapy, but they do not really know what to talk about. When I ask what they really desire in life beyond symptom reduction, they are unable to say. And when I ask what they want to get out of therapy, they get confused.

The topic of gender roles and gender relations arises in my own life as well. We seem to think about personal as well as social issues in gendered terms these days—I think we have to thank the women's movement for that development. Questions abound. What is manliness about? If it is about power, then what do we mean by power? Are material wealth, hierarchical status, and winning the "right woman" the only measures of power? How can a man compete to the best of his ability in the world of work if he has serious reservations about the ethics of a competitive life? How is a straight man who is striving not to be a sexist supposed to stand up to his wife or lover if it looks to him as if standing up to a woman could be interpreted as a sexist act? Are the issues very different for gay men?

The material for this book comes from my own life, my clinical experience, and my association with men in my family, friendships, men's groups, and more recently in men's conferences and gatherings. I write about clinical cases, among other things. Of course, I change names and details to insure confidentiality. And the discussion is not limited to clinical and psychotherapeutic issues. Rather, I use clinical material to illustrate the larger themes of gender, intimacy, and power in men's lives. I also write about my experiences and point out some links between my experiences and those of my friends and clients. Then I apply these experiences in a discussion of gender roles, gender relations, the men's movement, and the prospects for change.

Victor Seidler (1989) warns:

> It is important to recognize that at a level of personal experience and engagement in relationship, the invisibility to themselves that results from men's power and propensity to impersonalize and universalize their own experience tempt them into constantly talking for others, while presenting themselves as the neutral voices of reason. (p. 7)

The men I know best, and the men I treat in therapy, tend to be like me. A certain number are of different races, classes, and cultures; a minority are gay; but the majority are straight, white, and financially comfortable, like me. When I make comments that pertain exclusively to men like me, I risk leaving out gays, African-Americans, blue collar workers, and so forth. But if I include all men in my generalizations, I risk "talking for others."

The best way I know to handle this dilemma is to speak from my own experience, mention the limitations of that experience, and attempt to delineate the potential biases that are built into my observations. For instance, I know more about homophobia than I do about homosexuality. Without meaning to short-change gay men, I will concentrate more on homophobia in these pages. Meanwhile, with more open communication and collaboration between men and women, gay and straight, there is reason to hope that a collaborative look at these and other issues will begin to elicit a fair and comprehensive picture.

Discussions of masculinity and gender relations can be accompanied by pain and distress. Deborah Tannen (1990) points out a difficulty that regularly crops up:

> Some men hear any statement about women and men, coming from a woman, as an accusation—a fancy way of throwing up her hands, as if to say, "You Men!" They feel they are being objectified, if not slandered, by being talked about at all. (p. 14)

Because of this concern, many men hesitate to enter into discussions about masculinity and gender relations, even with other men, for fear they will be unfairly criticized. For instance, there is the notion that in our society men are in power, men oppress women, go to war, and destroy the environment, and therefore men are responsible for all that ails our civilization. While it is true that the people in power are almost all men, most men actually wield relatively little power, and though men are capable of violence against women and rape is omnipresent in our society, most men do not rape and I believe the majority feel deep respect for the women in their lives. In her study of the way men and women regularly misunderstand each other, Tannen does not concentrate on blaming men. Instead she tries to explain how the different assumptions that underlie men's and women's perceptions interfere with their attempts to communicate with each other.

As I write, there appears in the local newspaper (*Oakland Tribune*, June 1, 1991) a front page headline about vandals destroying a large statue of a goddess that was erected a few weeks earlier in the Emeryville mudflats along the East side of the San Francisco Bay. The artist, Jane Lowe, is quoted:

> The way it was mutilated reminds me of the way a lot of rapists act—they chopped the arms off, they chopped the hands off, they ripped the breasts off—You never hear about them doing that to boys.

My wife reads the article and turns to me, asking:

"Why do men hate women so?"

I think I understand what she is asking and begin to answer:

"Well, maybe they're angry at mothers who abused or neglected them, or maybe they're afraid of women who are independent and powerful like that artist or the goddess she sculpted."

Then I stop, realizing there is something wrong with this conversation. I, a man, would never vandalize a woman's sculpture. I understand men's feelings about powerful women because I occasionally feel threatened by powerful women, including my wife. But I don't hate women, would never attack a woman or her creative production, and, in fact, attempt at every oportunity to support women's rights, especially their right to be independent and powerful—and this means, of course, that I have to work through my intimidation each time it surfaces. So why am I explaining to my wife why "we" hate and attack "them?"

A distinction is needed, a distinction between men's occasional fantasies and private feelings and men's sexist or misogynist beliefs and actions. A man might be angry at his mother and unconsciously transfer that anger to the women in his adult life; that is a psychological problem many men are working through in their therapies. A man might secretly consume pornography that depicts women as sex objects while attempting, in real life, to treat women with respect as equals. The fact that unresolved anger toward his mother seeps into an interaction with a lover, or the consumption of pornography per se, does not make a man a misogynist.

Most of my friends and the men I see in therapy (the men I will write most about) would quite consciously disavow sexism. They believe that a woman has as much right as a man to work and be recognized for her successes, that a father has a responsibility to play a major role in childrearing, and they do not condone domestic violence, discrimination against gays and lesbians, date-rape, or sexual harassment. But it not always clear to them what constitutes sexism and homophobia, nor what nonsexist course of action might be available in any given situation. Besides, with gender relations undergoing radical change, the meaning of masculinity becomes blurred. While men are convinced they must still satisfy the requirements of the male role, they admit they are less and less certain what those requirements are. And they often feel falsely accused when some (but certainly not all) feminists and men who belong to the "pro-feminist" wing of the emerging men's movement make gross or inaccurate generalizations about the evils of all men.

Better, we might ask why men feel the way they do and how these feelings play a part in the pain and constrictions men experience. Then we can move on to a discussion of ways men might choose to be different. In the process, we will have to redefine power so that there can be a third alternative to the either/or, topdog/fallen subordinate schema we learned in the schoolyard, and men will not feel they must sacrifice their power in order to change for the better our notions about what it means to be a man, and to effect gender equality.

CHAPTER ONE

Nice Guys Needn't Finish Last

A large number of men believe that treating women as equals is the best way to attain not only a satisfying primary relationship but also personal fulfillment. They listen to women, learn from their demands and the way they live their lives, and work with them to end sexism at home as well as in society. Of course, the process is not always discussed in these terms. Many men would not link their respect for women at work or their equal participation in childrearing to the battle against sexism. But whether or not they think about it in terms of ending sexism, a generation of men learned in the 'sixties and 'seventies to do what had once been considered women's work: cooking, housecleaning, and childrearing, and they learned to work alongside women, and treat them with respect.

If the venture was at all successful, they also learned that there are payoffs to the redivision of labor, including the joys of close contact with children from infancy, the experience of sharing feelings, the opportunity to admit weaknesses and ask for help in relationships that permit mutual dependency, and relief from the pressure to always be the strong shoulder to lean on, the one capable of fixing a woman's every problem. At the same time these men learned what it means to really respect a woman's right to realize her full power in the world at large, and that there are benefits for men in a more equal arrangement.

Men who came of age after the 'sixties movements waned never had the opportunity to be involved in the struggles of those days, but their lives have been deeply affected by women's social gains. Women have been admitted to previously all-male colleges and universities and men are attending academies that were established for women only. Women are entering jobs and professions previously reserved for men and working their way up the hierarchy. Dianne Ehrensaft (1987) chronicles the attempts of a large number of dual-career couples to share equally the burdens and joys of childrearing. Meanwhile men are taking on more of the jobs that were once considered women's work, from toilet-cleaning and childrearing to secretarial work and nursing.

Judith Stacey (1990) examines the ramifications of feminism among working class families in California's Silicon Valley, pointing out that though these men and women do not acknowledge the effects of feminism and are not social activists, their lives have been deeply affected by the women's movement. Stacey comments about the young adult women she interviewed:

> Ignorant or disdainful of the political efforts feminists expended to secure such gains, they are preoccupied instead coping with the expanded opportunities and burdens women now encounter. (p. 264)

Stacey also comments about the men:

> Almost all of the men I observed or heard about routinely performed tasks that my own blue-collar father and his friends never deigned to contemplate .... Although the division of household labor remains profoundly inequitable, I am convinced that a major gender norm has shifted here. (p. 268)

This phenomenon is not limited to Silicon Valley. Gender relations are in flux. More women are assuming positions of power in the public sphere and more men support women's efforts while assuming more of the burdens of domestic life.

For a while it did seem to many that the idealism of the 'sixties could live on in the personal attempts to attain equality between the sexes. But then mishaps began to occur. Relationships floundered. Illness, the deaths of loved ones, or the failure to achieve the aims of one's life threw many men into emotional turmoil. Men who were unable to find satisfying work or lost opportunities for promotion saw women getting more jobs and more promotions, including the women they were personally supporting.

Men tired of hearing the many ways they were guilty of sexism, they could not stand to hear once again what is wrong with men, and they began to suspect that the women in their lives were utilizing the charge of sexism to enhance their power in heterosexual relationships.

Some began to feel that, while women had support groups and an audience as they talked incessantly about the need to empower women, there were few if any opportunities for men to talk about their problems and insecurities. In addition there was the accusation that men who attend too closely to women's needs and desires are "Momma's boys," "soft males," and "wimps." Many men began to realize that being supportive of women's struggles was not enough.

The men I am describing are ambivalent about power. On the one hand, they do not want to act the brute, compete ruthlessly at work and dominate at home in order to demonstrate their adequacy as men; on the other hand, when they pull back from the cutthroat competition in the public arena and support women's power at the expense of their own at work and at home, they end up feeling powerless, manipulated, and inadequate. These men would like to discover ways to be powerful without being sexist, and ways to stop obsessing about the theme of power and men's place in an oppressive hierarchy.

Jim

Jim entered my office nervously and walked around, looking at the art on the walls and the books on the shelves. He smiled, as if pleased, and sat down, sinking slowly into a semifetal position on the chair as he began to speak:

"My wife is having an affair. I don't know what to do. I'm so jittery I can't sleep nights. Do I tell her I know and start a big fight—maybe break us up—or do I just shut up about it, treat her well, and hope she'll stop seeing the guy?"

After a few minutes he began to cry, apologizing and saying he has not cried like this in years.

"I've done everything right. We always negotiated every decision we made together, and I always made sure we were divvying things up equally. Now she's cheating on me, treating me like dirt. And this guy she's seeing—a real sleaze—he doesn't even know what feminism is all about! It just isn't fair!"

By now he was speaking angrily, sitting up in his chair and urgently leaning toward me.

Jim had always supported his wife's efforts to succeed and feel powerful. They met in the 'seventies. She was in a women's consciousness-raising group. He was very interested in what she was learning about herself. They married and he supported her while she returned to university to earn a graduate degree in a professional school. After she graduated and established herself in her profession, they had two children. Following each birth he cut back at work and did much of the housework while she returned to part-time work within a few months.

Jim always thought they had an ideal relationship. What went wrong? We talked quite a bit about this. His wife had grown up with a strict and critical father who would not permit her much freedom as a girl. She chose for a mate someone who listened to her, made her feel self-assured, and helped her to be very much her own person. Jim had learned from an early age to put his needs aside and take care of his depressed mother—this was the only way he could feel close to her—and was therefore ready and able to "take care of" his wife in many very admirable ways. They were both psychologically prepared for the message of the women's movement and sincerely attempted to put it into practice in their everyday lives. They spent fifteen years together.

Being treated well, she enjoyed her newfound freedom for awhile. She developed confidence. Then she began to feel there was something wrong. Perhaps she could not put it into words, and needed to emote or act out in seemingly irrational ways—by screaming at him without reason or by having an affair. He, meanwhile, was not very good at setting limits with the person he most wanted to please. So she felt unmet, out of control, or just plain irritable. He felt for some time that she was not very interested in satisfying his needs, but he said nothing about this.

Jim's marriage needed a serious overhaul, and each of the partners needed to look at his or her own personal issues. We discussed the situation, examined Jim's inability to confront his wife, and related his limitations to some still unprocessed conflicts he had about his early relationship with his mother. He defended his mother—as if talking about her faults constituted disloyalty—but then became aware of a certain amount of resentment he had always harbored toward her. He began to see he had been suppressing similar resentment toward his wife, resentment that had been mounting long before she began the affair. Soon after commencing therapy, Jim decided to stop crying silently and fading into the furniture. He confronted his wife, told her he knew about the affair, and for once expressed more outrage than she during a heated battle that resulted in their sleeping in separate rooms for several nights.

He considered leaving her at this point and, by his account, she considered leaving him. In the end, neither wanted to end the relationship. She promised to stop seeing her lover, and they decided to see a therapist together and renew their efforts to make the marriage work. Meanwhile, he began his own psychotherapy in earnest, the primary goal being to feel more self-confident, more "manly"—without giving up his commitment to equality between the sexes.

A Certain Lack of Vitality

Psychoanalysis has taught us to look for personal constrictions in three general areas: love, work, and play. In all three areas the men I am describing regularly report feeling a lack of power and vitality. Many are unable to stand up to a woman just when they both need him to. If he continually attends to his partner's needs and remains quiet about the fact she is not as interested in attending to his, he either builds up resentment that has no outlet until he develops an ulcer or has an affair, or he becomes timid and depressed, fearing that any other response would threaten the stability of the relationship—perhaps he fears the repercussions of the rage that is building inside. Or the man's lack of vitality might be reflected in his inability to come forth with his feelings and desires.

Alternatively, the single man's difficulties finding a partner might be related to the idea that, once he commits himself to a relationship, the partner will gain control of him and he will lose his personal freedom as well as his sense of identity. There is a kernel of truth, as usual: If he does not learn to be clear about his feelings and desires, she will always seem to him to be in control of their relationship and he will wind up feeling he is passively reacting to her moods.

Quite a few single men seek therapy mainly because they believe there is something wrong with them, causing their relationships to go awry. They, like men who are in long-term relationships and encourage their partners to be powerful, must get past this dilemma if their relationships are to be sound and lasting. For instance, a single man recently consulted me following the break-up of a year long romantic relationship with a woman that had been "a disaster" for him. He quickly identified the problem: from the start he had let the woman make all the decisions; she began to despise him for his weakness and treat him cruelly, for instance telling friends about his problem with premature ejaculation; and when he complained about her cruelty there were loud and vicious arguments.

"I was left with the choice of screaming at her or getting out, so I got out."

He told me he has resolved to prevent a repetition of that traumatic episode by avoiding women altogether. We began to explore the reasons he did not believe he might, in future relationships, insist from the beginning on establishing trust and making half the decisions, and in the process find a partner who would be willing to share power more equally.

Ted's wife was first attracted to him because of his "softness." He had grown up in a home that was organized around his father's tyrannical style. Ted's father would yell at Ted's mother whenever she missed a step—burned dinner or failed to respond to a child's frantic call from school, making him interrupt an important meeting in order to ferry a sick child home. He wonders if his father's constant complaints about his mother might have been his father's reaction to her disinterest in sex. He will never know. But his father was a tyrant, and he swore from an early age never to be anything like him. He always respected his wife's right to carry on a life of her own, with professional activities and numerous intimacies.

"The only problem," he adds with sadness in his eyes, "is that now she's saying I don't stand up for myself enough."

Because of continuing squabbles Ted and his wife go to see a marriage therapist. After a few sessions she tells them that she thinks the problem is insufficient emotional contact between the two of them, and that his wife seems to miss it more than Ted does—so, his wife quite often starts fights with Ted in order to create emotional contact. Fighting is better than no contact at all. This has been true of their relationship from the beginning, what has changed is that she can no longer tolerate his lack of strength in the ensuing fights. She needs him to stand up to her so that she can figure out where her boundaries end and his begin. Without that, she feels very out-of-control, sometimes crazy.

Ted cannot figure out whether he should get tougher—that is, be more like his father—or keep giving in to his wife in their arguments, for instance doing what she says now and fighting harder. Isn't giving in to his wife in this argument—by getting tougher with her, thereby giving her precisely what she wants—just another sign of weakness? I raise the possibility he might insist she begin to appreciate the ways in which he already demonstrates his toughness—for instance, how avidly he supports her professional life and her right to maintain close intimacies with women friends, even though he often feels left out when she is out doing exciting things with others. My job is to help Ted begin to believe that a man might assert himself within a heterosexual relationship without becoming a brute, and, alternatively, that he can occasionally bow to his wife's wishes without seeing himself as a weakling.

Often a couple's problems surface in the emotional turmoil of one or more of their children. For instance, the father—whether living with the mother or divorced—might make a habit of bowing to the mother's will, leaving the child to experience his father as passive or absent and his mother as controlling. There are many reasons why a father might bow in this way; his passivity might be characterological, it might be grounded in early interactions with a controlling mother, he might be afraid of his wife's wrath or abandonment if he asserts himself, or, in the case of a divorce where the father left the mother, his passivity might be an expression of the guilt he feels for breaking up the family. The man's inability to express his power with women is passed on as a problem to another generation. Sons find their fathers' weakness and passivity disappointing, and report feeling they lack a role model. One of the positive ramifications of the emergence of a men's movement (and renewed interest in male psychology) is that fathers are figuring out new ways to be strong. The model of parents resolving their differences as equals without resorting to distancing or abusiveness makes it possible for the children to envision a relationship based on mutual respect, and there is no reason a healthy relationship of this kind cannot develop between divorced parents as well.

The lack of vitality in the work arena is often less visible, the man being competent enough, and complaining little about his dissatisfactions. Only when problems get entirely out of hand—for instance with a business failure, bankruptcy, layoff, or stress-induced ulcer—only then do these men consult a therapist about their conflicts about work. They tend to be quite bright and talented, and, on the surface at least, seem to have achieved quite a bit in their lives. But on closer examination it becomes apparent they have not achieved all that they might, or all they might wish. It turns out they have been holding themselves back. They have always used their talents to succeed just enough to support a family or attain a modicum of recognition from their peers, but they have not applied themselves fully to any ambitious project. Again, the most notable symptom of their malaise is a certain lack of vigor, or competitive edge.

Harold, an attorney, had spent his first few years out of law school as an associate in a "high-power, prestigious firm." He did not mind working sixty hours per week as much as he minded what he terms the "ass-licking/ass-kicking mentality" that was required of those who wished to become partners in the firm. But at the same time he felt that attorneys who worked on their own and did less important cases were not serious about the law. Eventually he left the firm and did some criminal defense work. But there he felt he could never do a satisfactory job preparing a defense, the work load being so overwhelming and the public defender's budget so limited. He reports:

"I burned out on that and went into solo practice."

There he ended up doing "the kind of unimportant cases I used to criticize others for taking."

By the time he began psychotherapy he was very depressed, bored at work, unable to figure out any changes he might make, and kicking himself about the trajectory of his career.

For many men it is the third area, play, that is the most problematic. It is also the lowest priority. Some men, especially those with a busy career and young children at home, state categorically that they have no time to play. Others, single or with careers firmly established, who have no children or whose children are older and more independent, complain they have forgotten how to play. Even when they are athletic, their demanding workouts and athletic contests seem more like work than play, and they lack friends. At least they express some nostalgia about their teens and college years when, as one client recently told me:

"It was easier back then, there were guys I hung out with and we just did things together—now I wouldn't know what to do, and the men I know are all too busy with work and families to just hang out."

These men link their inability to play with their lack of friends:

"There is no one to play with."

Alex tells me his father was essentially absent—he suspects he had many affairs—and his mother was very dependent on him, the oldest child. She would drink Scotch, go to bed, turn off the lights, and cry for hours. He always needed to reassure his younger siblings. Then, when they quieted down, he would go see if there was anything he could do to make his mother feel better. Or, if his father returned, he would take his brother and two sisters out of the house and give his parents some privacy and time to work things out. Meanwhile, he had to help his siblings with their homework, do his chores, and do his own homework—all of which he did so well that he won a full scholarship to a prestigious college.

Alex is successful in his profession and has a family of his own now. But he is still unable to let go, to really enjoy himself. He tells me he never relaxes at social events, he is always worried lest someone not have a good time. And he is unable to take time for himself, so worried is he that there's someone he should be checking on. Of course, the pattern has been there from childhood. He took care of the whole family as a child. That is a very big job for a small boy, a job that would hasten maturity if he were to accomplish it, and would make him ever vigilant lest he fall down on the job. When the boy is unable to play, the man has no childhood play experience to fall back on. Worse, the man carries on the child's sense of the current task as overwhelming, in spite of an adult life full of evidence that this man is more than a match for almost any task, and that the most important tasks—for instance the attainment of success at work and a happy family life—have already been accomplished. The man's inner sense of an ominously large burden resists revision. And one cannot figure out how to play by utilizing serious, rational exercises. In fact, Alex is unable to play precisely because he is too serious about the project of figuring out how to play. As D.W. Winnicott (1971) advises, Alex and I need to "play" in the consulting room so that he can learn to duplicate the experience in his life outside of therapy.

Men Who Abhor Domination

Why do some men support gender equality while others do not? Many experts on male psychology blame an overly involved mother for the adult male's inability to stand up to a woman, his underachievement at work, and his general lack of vitality (Olsen, 1981). Others blame passive or absent fathers (Biller, 1970; Carvalho, 1982). In his popular book, *Passive Men, Wild Women*, Pierre Mornell (1979) blames both. According to Mornell, the man's mother was immensely disappointed in his absent, abusive, or weak father:

> The disappointed mother—and this was the crucial point—then transferred her expectations from the husband to the son. Not only did she transfer her expectations, but also her sexual energy—once directed toward the husband and marriage—was now poured into her son . . . . Her boy became the primary focus of her adoration and expectations. (p. 47)

Of course there are cases where the man was overly involved with his mother, perhaps the one in the family who was most attuned to her needs and most interested in taking care of her. Sometimes he was the one who was "special" in her eyes, the one she could adore while she continually devalued her husband. Tom, played by Nick Nolte in *The Prince of Tides*, reports to his sister's psychiatrist that his mother told him he was so special that she loved him the most, and that he only found out years later that she had told both his brother and sister the same thing. There are many histories of physically or emotionally absent fathers, or abusive ones, or overly critical ones. But quite a few of the men I am describing report that they were not particularly close with their mothers and that they had a fairly close relationship with a father who was capable of nurturing others and treating women as equals. Or they report that they were not close with either parent. In other words, there is no single pattern in the background of all these men. It is amazing how some men who were abused or neglected by both parents evolved the capacity to be intimate and attain sexual equalty. It is as if, while they were being abused, they were imagining how things might be different and vowing never to make anyone else suffer the way they suffered. I have heard from several men in therapy that this was indeed the case, and that they remember how much better they felt as children when they concentrated very hard on that vow while enduring repeated abuse.

My own impression in working with these men is that they do not all spring from one Oedipal constellation or share a particular type of personality or psychopathology. After all, psychoanalysts have been notably unsuccessful in their efforts to uncover a generalizable theory on the etiology of homosexuality (Friedman, 1986). Aside from the fact that their approach has been riddled with unexplored homophobic biases, there just does not seem to be one story that fits all gay men. Rather, there are many idiosyncratic personal stories. Similarly, there is no single early precursor of support for gender equality in men.

These men do share one important attribute: an early acquired abhorrence for relationships based on domination, particularly with regard to gender relations. There seems to be a lifelong wish for a relationship of mutuality (Benjamin, 1988).

If there is no single childhood scenario that explains why it is very important to certain men to treat women with respect, perhaps we can begin to understand the psychology of these men by assuming there is a range of tolerance for domination in human relationships. The range is obvious in a family where the father is abusive. One child will stand up to the father, perhaps to protect the mother, another will cower, while a third might identify with the abusive father. Perhaps the difference is related to birth order, perhaps to temperament, perhaps to the mother's choice of a champion from among the children. There are many relevant variables, each worthy of exploration in individual cases. But it is difficult to identify a single explanation of the reactions of all children in this or any other kind of family scenario. Similarly, the early family dramas of these men can involve a nurturing father and a loving parental dyad, and one son can grow up to be quite traditional while another becomes a champion of gender equality. There is no simple formula.

If a child grows up believing something that is contrary to the explicit belief system of his family or culture, if he is not sufficiently articulate to put his beliefs into words nor sure enough of himself to espouse his belief system in any forceful way, and if, when he lives out his beliefs, he receives admonitions or worried glances from those around him, then he develops doubts about himself. Many of the men I am describing have had this kind of experience. Perhaps as a child in a family that fostered competitiveness and ambition in boys, he was less interested in competing and rising to the top than he was in being close to others and attending to their feelings. Stories vary here. Sometimes the boy's mother supported his interest in interpersonal relationships while his father railed on about his lack of manliness and ambition. Sometimes the parents were both ambivalent about ambition, giving the child mixed messages about the importance of striving for excellence. A client recently told me that his leftist parents were both ambivalent about success, feeling that most successful people had "sold out" somewhere along the way. The parents passed their ambivalence on to their child, who at age 24 complains he has been unable to get started in any particular career track.

If the boy's beliefs did not clash with his family's, he might have come to grief when faced with the schoolyard drama where he was forced to fight or be called chicken. Perhaps he had no interest in fighting but was unable to find a third alternative. Or perhaps as a teenager he was repulsed by the prospect of bragging to other boys about his sexual conquests and divulging names and details of acts committed—Jim remembers being deeply troubled when his male friends in high school began devaluing women in this way. Sensitive men regularly report doubts about themselves that they trace to early experiences where they felt very much the oddball for refusing to posture "like a man."

The initiation of boys into teen peer culture often includes humiliation, where the humiliated newcomer is permitted and expected to regain his sense of composure and belonging by turning around and joining the other boys in humiliating the next newcomer who happens along. Thus Steve, now in his early forties, tells me that he was picked to play on a regional select baseball team at age 14. Most of the boys on the team were older, and he was the only one who joined the team in the middle of the season. After the first practice, when he went into the locker room to shower, his teammates jumped him, stripped him naked, and while three held him down the others pinched his torso until he was black and blue, meanwhile making nasty cracks about his "baby fat" and the small size of his genitals. Then they let him go and nothing more was ever said about the incident. When, at the beginning of the following season, it became clear his teammates were planning to initiate two new team members in similar fashion, and would mock him if he did not participate, Steve quit the team. He confesses I am the only person he has ever told about the incident.

Peggy Reeves Sanday (1990) describes in graphic detail the kind of humiliation that occurs when certain college fraternities initiate their "pledges"—including stripping the pledges and mocking their genitals, putting them in diapers, and calling them girls. Then, these young men become members and join their "brothers" in doing the same things to the next group of pledges. Because her source of data is interviews she conducted with fraternity members, Sanday does not mention the young men who never pledged fraternities and would never take part in such cruel rituals, nor does she mention the many men who did take part but later regretted the cruel acts they committed as youngsters. Men who refused to participate in the teen rituals often report that they felt very isolated at that stage of development.

Max, a building tradesman who grew up in a working class family, complains he lacks confidence in social situations, particularly with women, and this is why, at age 29, he has never had a satisfactory sexual relationship, not to mention a long-term intimacy. As a teenager he felt isolated. He wanted to be more social, but believed others did not like him. I ask why and he explains he was not interested in the things other kids were interested in.

"All the guys wanted to talk about was sports and girls—and I didn't like the way they talked about girls—I had two sisters and I didn't want any guys talking about them in a disgusting way."

Listening to Max, I found myself reminiscing silently about my own teen years. In high school girls I liked told me they really valued our friendship, I was "so sensitive" and easy to talk to, and I would be "just the kind of guy" they would like to marry someday, but for the time being they were more interested in dating a different kind of guy, in other words a more exciting one such as the high school quarterback, the biker, or the college fratman.

I had to force myself to snap out of my reminiscing and figure out what to say to Max. I decided to say approximately what I would have liked an older man to say to me when I was struggling with some of the same issues:

"Sensitive men often have trouble as teenagers. High school culture values tough-guy-ness. Guys regularly say disrespectful things about girls, I think it might be an attempt for them to bolster their sense of manliness. So a sensitive guy who doesn't want to talk that way has a hard time. But later, as an adult, the same sensitivity can turn out to be a very valuable asset. It can make men better at whatever they do, and women value it in a way they were not able to admit in high school. Their part of the high school game is to admire the tough guy who puts women down. Maybe they have unresolved conflicts about a brutish father. When they get a little older they might figure out it's much better to hook up with a man who can be sensitive to their needs and treat them with respect. The challenge for a sensitive man like you is to weather the high school rejections and not give up the sensitivity. Then, a bunch of years later, that sensitivity is one of the things others will find most lovable about you."

Max cried a little at the end of that session. In the weeks that followed he broke off a relationship with a woman who consumed large quantities of alcohol and refused to listen to him when he demanded she stop. He decided not to date for awhile, at least until he figured out why he always chose women who were self-destructive and refused to listen to him. Of course we linked this question to his relationship with his mother. But a part of the psychodynamics here had to do with revenge for insults suffered in high school. He chose women with tough exteriors, the kind who might have dated the football captain in high school, then he uncovered their fatal flaws—for instance alcoholism—and was able to feel superior while taking care of them. Several months passed before he met a woman who was very different, the woman he eventually married. She was very strong, yet interested in what he had to say.

Another male client in his early forties seeks therapy because he feels he is not "getting very far" in his career and lacks ambition. He tells me his father was very ambitious and describes the older man's talents and status in the business world. I point out how proud he seems of his father and ask why it is so hard to emulate him. He answers that his father was an alcoholic and very abusive toward his mother. He always took his mother's side. He remembers his father raging and pushing his mother out the bedroom door. With tears he begins to explore a fantasy he had as a child but had forgotten: that all powerful men are abusive at home.

The Male Theme

In my clinical work with men, spanning twenty years, I have been impressed by the omnipresence of a single theme: Men view themselves, consciously or unconsciously, as at the top or the bottom of some hierarchy—and, if at the top, needing always to remain vigilant lest they fall or be thrown to the bottom. The man on top is successful, powerful, virile, admirable, heroic, lovable, and so on. At the bottom he is weak, humiliated, impotent, shunned, cowardly, and despised—a failure. There is a rigid either/or quality to the theme, the man feeling at times there is no third alternative.

This theme occurs in men's fantasies; it also reflects an aspect of our social reality. Christopher Lasch (1979), among others, points out that our "culture of narcissism" fosters this theme in men. Robert Bellah and his collaborators (1985) link the problem to the American male's obsession with individualism and self-sufficiency. This is not to say all men view their plight in just these terms, nor that all men are obsessed with power and domination. Rather, the theme is present to some extent in the male psyche, and each man must work out his own way of relating to the theme as it surfaces periodically in his life. The sensitive, nontraditional man is no exception.

Women are not immune to the male theme, of course. Naomi Wolf (1991) explains that acceptance of "the beauty myth," including the notion that there is a universal standard for judging a woman's beauty, leads women to collude with men in maintaining the male theme. By worrying about their relative beauty, women "keep male dominance intact." According to Wolf:

> In assigning value to women in a vertical hierarchy according to a culturally imposed physical standard, it is an expression of power relations in which women must unnaturally compete for resources that men have appropriated for themselves. (p. 12)

It is no accident that women who are challenging men's obsession with hierarchies are also challenging women's obsession with media-dictated standards of female beauty.

Michael Maccoby (1976), having interviewed a large number of successful male corporate managers, has this to say about them:

> He wants to be known as a winner, and his deepest fear is to be labelled a loser . . . . He tries to use the company for his own ends, fearing that otherwise he will be totally emasculated by the corporation. (p. 100)

Aren't most men terrified of being dominated? Perhaps it takes the form of a business failure, loss of a competitive battle at work or in sports, loss of a woman to another man, or merely the possibility someone might stab one in the back. The tendency for men to cannibalize each other is socially constructed and deeply internalized in the male psyche.

The theme is omnipresent in American literature. Consider Theodore Dreiser's (1900) classic novel, *Sister Carrie*. Carrie's second lover, Hurstwood, is the successful manager of a fashionable club when they meet. He proceeds to steal from the club, deceive his wife about his infidelity, and lie to Carrie. By the end of the novel, he and Carrie have moved from Chicago to New York, broken up, she has become a star on Broadway, and he has sunk to ever new lows of poverty and unemployment. Eventually they meet on the street outside her theater, where he is begging for a handout. Here is the underside of the American dream, the ideal being the "self-made man." If everyone has the opportunity to become rich and famous, then those who fail in their quest have only themselves to blame. The man on the bottom thinks of himself as deeply flawed, and others become workaholics for fear they will fall to the bottom.

Of course the parts for the adult drama are learned at home and at school. At home the boy learns about the pecking order, about the father's authority, the mother's submission and the child's smallness and inability to change the family hierarchy. Freud conceptualized the theme of hierarchy in terms of the penis. The boy has one, the girl does not. The boy discovers this fact during his second year and draws two conclusions: he is somehow privileged in relation to the girl, and her lack means castration is possible (Freud, 1925). In addition, the boy's penis is small, the father's large. Thus the boy finds his place in the hierarchy: possession of a penis gives him higher status than females, but the size of his penis means lower status in relation to another male, his father. This is Freud's formulation. Karen Horney (1924, 1926, 1935), Clara Thompson (1942, 1943) and other pioneer psychoanalysts moved away from Freud's phallocentrism, pointing out that possession of a penis is a way for men to rationalize their domination and not a biological given, and male domination is something that can be changed. Since the late 'sixties feminist psychoanalysts, including Nancy Chodorow (1978) and Dorothy Dinnerstein (1976), have attempted to free Freud's Oedipal formulation from its sexist biases. Freud's is not the only explanation of the way hierarchy is learned at home. Still, home is where the lessons begin.

At school the lessons are refined and reinforced (Connell, 1989). According to Jules Henry (1963), the gradeschooler learns that for someone to succeed, someone else must fail. Henry relates the story of an observer he sent to an elementary school classroom as part of his research in urban anthropology. The observer watched as Boris stood at the blackboard and looked at a math problem. Boris could not figure out the answer. The teacher suggested he "think!" Boris' mind was still a blank. By this time there were several hands waving in the classroom. Several classmates were having trouble staying in their seats, so excited were they about the prospect of Boris failing to figure out the answer and the teacher calling on them. Henry comments:

> This is the standard condition of the American elementary school, and is why so many of us feel a contraction of the heart even if someone we never knew succeeds merely at garnering plankton in the Thames: because so often somebody's success has been bought at the cost of our failure. (p.296).

The male theme stands out boldly in psychosis. Consider the manic episode that follows a man's fall from a position of power into bankruptcy. Rather than feeling depressed about his plight, he manufactures the delusional belief that the bankruptcy was for the best and he need not seek employment because he is soon to be selected CEO of a large corporation. Thus, he explains in a cheerful tone, there is no cause for sadness. Another man, paranoid, compensates for his severe sense of inadequacy by imagining that dozens of undercover FBI agents have been assigned to follow him and tap his phone—as if he were that important. In both cases, the man believes he has fallen to the bottom of the heap and compensates with a delusional sense of power and importance.

In the more typical case it is only after a certain amount of self-exploration that a relatively healthy and functional man discovers the theme in his unconscious. For instance, a man came to my office for a consultation complaining of deep depression. He told me he was a "workaholic" and no longer wished to be—but when he stopped working, even for a short vacation, he became very anxious. Meanwhile his wife was threatening to leave him because he was never around. We eventually discovered that the anxiety was related to an unconscious fantasy: "If I don't keep working every waking hour I will be beaten by envious competitors and fail miserably at my job." Of course the fantasy also contained the idea that, once beaten, his wife would definitely abandon him.

The either/or-ness of the theme is reflected in a series of polarities: big/small; strong/weak; success/failure; lovable/despicable. The last is very familiar to anyone who has ever fallen from the heights of love to the depths of self-doubt after being left by the loved one. The first is just as well known, the big/small pair being central to this society's male culture. There is the lore of penis size: the jokes, the boys with bigger ones making fun of those with smaller ones, the fear of being unable to satisfy a woman because one's penis is too small—a fear that is aggravated by porno magazines where male protagonists are always "well hung." We cannot befriend each other for fear of being betrayed in a dog-eat-dog world, we use women to prop up our sense of potency, we hate illness and cannot stand the aging process because of our dread of vulnerability and failure. Helen Caldicott (1984) links the threat of nuclear annihilation with the male theme, pointing to the "missile envy" that keeps the world on the verge of war. The either/or quality is so intense that a man who feels like a loser in any one regard feels like a loser in all regards—small, weak, a failure, and unlovable.

Nice Guys Must Cope with the Male Theme, Too

I have noticed a pattern in the way a large number of men handle this theme. Realizing at a very early age that they did not want to play either role, these men remember always trying to pull back just a little from engagement in male games and male posturing, biding their time and trying to find a path that would not require them to be either victor or vanquished. They always had sufficient abilities—athletic, intellectual, creative, or social—to get by, and as long as they did not push themselves as much as they might to excel or to reach the very top, they were able to walk a line somewhere between the insensitive posturing man and the weak, submissive loser. But having pulled back from the male drama of the schoolyard, the mating game, the beer hall, the fraternity, or the board room just enough to avoid having to play one of the two polar roles, they found there was no strong role left for them. They eventually experienced low self-esteem or a worrisome lack of vitality; the former because they, like all males, have internalized the male theme to a significant extent and feel like losers; the latter because, in pulling back from the male drama, they have had to suppress a certain amount of the passion that is typically called forth by competitive male pursuits, and that kind of suppression has become something of a habit.

I do not mean to imply that disdain for domination was always conscious. Jim did not view his submissiveness in these terms; Harold never verbalized his conflicts about ambition until after he graduated from law school; and Steve always wondered if he was "less of a man" for refusing to participate in his baseball team's cruel initiation ritual. In their early years most of these men were not sufficiently formed as autonomous individuals to design alternative roles for themselves. And boys who were having the same difficulty were unable to support each other at that time because they, too, believed "real men" just did not discuss with each other their doubts about being a man.

In many cases, these men found some respite in the arms of a woman during young adulthood. There are many versions of the story. In Rilke's (1912, 1989) version, the prodigal son leaves home because he cannot "stay and conform to this lying life of approximations which they have assigned to him, and come to resemble them all in every feature of his face." Instead, he would "love again and again in his solitude, each time squandering his whole nature and in unspeakable fear for the freedom of the other person." Each time he fell in love, "he was now once again overcome by the growing urgency of his heart. And this time he hoped to be answered. His whole being, which during his long solitude had become prescient and imperturbable, promised him that the one he was now turning to would be capable of loving with a penetrating, radiant love." Eventually, the prodigal son returns home, "For he had lost hope of ever mating the woman whose love could pierce him." Like Rilke and his prodigal son, some men never find a woman whose love will pierce them and set them free. Others are more successful in their quest. But flight into a woman's arms does not provide lasting resolution of a man's conflicts, especially his conflicts about the male theme.

Reframing Childhood Memories

When, as adults, these men encountered women who were demanding equality, respect and an end to sexual exploitation, a resonant chord was struck deep within them. It was not only the obvious fairness of gender equality; finally there was external validation for what had been an all too private struggle to find a tenable stance as a man that did not require one to oppress others or be seen as a weakling or a loser. These men could understand their lifelong ambivalence about power, male posturing, and ambition in relation to an explicit theory of domination. Like an interpretation given in therapy, this adult understanding permitted a man to reconstruct childhood memories— of schoolyard fights or failure to be accepted by male peers because of a refusal to tell sex stories about girls—and this time see himself as a small, unsung hero. And now he would gain women's support for being among those rare men who were sensitive and not sexist—the very qualities that had led to derision from other boys in earlier years.

Family therapists speak of "reframing" events, putting them in a better light that permits the participants to maintain their dignity or feel loved by others with whom they interact in irrational ways. In the introduction I discussed my reframing of George's dilemma. He felt inadequate because his wife's salary exceeded his, and I pointed out that without his willingness to share childrearing responsibilities his wife would not be able to succeed as she has at work, and it was only because of his commitment to equal responsibilities at home that he was unable to work longer hours at the office and earn a promotion. George's depression occurred because he was trapped in the either/or theme. I offered him a third alternative, a way to view his principled commitment to equal coparenting as a powerful stance instead of a loser's excuse. As a therapist I find myself continually reframing men's stories, redefining power, and giving them an opportunity to see how powerful they are in spite of their failure to climb all the way to the top of traditional hierarchies.

But life goes on, and the hero of one day is not necessarily a hero the next. Women were very happy to find men who respected them as equals and were willing to change their ways. That happiness, however, eventually wore thin. The women continued to build their movement, and feminism evolved in new directions, women meeting with each other in various contexts to improve their lot and struggle collectively. What about the men? There is still very little support available for men who relate best to women and eschew traditional male competition and posturing. Friendships among men remain problematic. And men have less capability than women to get together with each other and strategize about the next step, let alone satisfy their needs for intimacy.

The man who goes against the tide is doubly isolated. He is isolated from traditional male circles where he is viewed as less than manly. But there are a large number of men who feel uncomfortable in traditional male circles. The problem is their difficulty getting together and supporting each other. Many say that they find it easier to be alone or to relate on an emotional level exclusively with women. Thus these men, enough like traditional heterosexual men to be hesitant about forming close, same-sex intimacies, are left out of traditional male circles while being relatively inept at forming alternative networks. The emerging men's movement is a real cause for hope here, as is the new resolve on the part of a large number of men to improve their intimacies with other men and to achieve a new level of equality and connectedness with women.

CHAPTER TWO

Pathological Arrhythmicity in Men

Premenstrual syndrome (PMS) is upsetting the professional equilibrium of the American Psychiatric Association. APA members are debating whether to include PMS as a diagnostic category in the forthcoming revised edition of the Association's *Diagnostic and Statistical Manual of Mental Disorders* (Spitzer, Severino, Williams, & Parry, 1989). The official title for the syndrome is late luteal phase dysphoric disorder—the luteal phase of the menstrual cycle denoting the time from ovulation to menses; dysphoria meaning a state of feeling unwell. Feminists argue that including PMS on psychiatry's official list of mental disorders would be just one more opportunity for men to pathologize the experience of women. Hilary Allen (1984) argues against utilizing premenstrual tension as a basis for establishing diminished capacity in legal proceedings because, if women were viewed as suffering from a hormone-based mental condition, then all women would be seen by the law as "close to madness and prone to crime." Amid much debate, the APA decided to leave this diagnostic category out of the revised third edition of the manual (American Psychiatric Association, 1987), but to include a description of late luteal phase dysphoric disorder in the appendix—leaving open the possibility of declaring it an official category later.

Of course, from a traditional male perspective, women are overly responsive to natural cycles. For instance, there is the familiar story of the woman being considered for a job or a promotion, only to be rejected when the male boss concludes that women are not as reliable as men—they take more sick days, they are more likely to quit when they get married, they require maternity leave, and they can be emotionally unpredictable, particularly at certain times of the month. This kind of gender discrimination is built into official hearings and court proceedings regarding rape, sexual harassment, and sex between male psychiatrists and female patients. Besides the fact that his past sexual history is often not admissible while hers is, when the woman contradicts herself in the midst of an emotional display her emotionality is viewed—mostly by males—as evidence that her story does not hold up, while the man's calm demeanor and extremely logical telling and reframing of his story are accepted as a believable defense.

Sometimes the woman is so articulate her claims cannot be dismissed. Dr. Frances Conley, a neurosurgeon and Professor in the Department of Surgery at Stanford Medical School, resigned from the faculty protesting rampant sexism. She explained:

> As a fellow faculty member, I felt I had the right to express an honest difference of opinion but found any deviation from the majority view often was announced prominently as a manifestation of either PMS or being "on the rag." I find myself unwilling to be called "hon" or "honey" with the same degree of sweet condescension used by this department for all women. (*San Francisco Chronicle*, June 4, 1991)

She was later asked to withdraw her resignation and she did, after the department agreed to take steps to end sexual harassment.

Can it be a coincidence that just when a large number of women are proving themselves to be very competent in responsible positions of formerly male privilege, that a new category of mental disorder, reserved for women, finds its way onto the psychiatric profession's official list?

The Male Equivalent

The male counterpart to late luteal phase dysphoric disorder is pathological arrhythmicity. Before anyone turns to the *Diagnostic and Statistical Manual* to look it up, I should mention that I am inventing this category of mental disorder as I write. In contrast to women, men suffer from too little responsiveness to natural cycles—in fact to cycles of any kind. The coping styles we have evolved in order to succeed at work—working long hours without letting up, arriving at work each day even when not feeling well, hiding our true feelings, remaining vigilant before the prospect of attack from as-yet-undisclosed enemies—all depend on our ability to override natural cycles. It is natural to cry when hurt and laugh raucously when something appears very funny; thus, our practiced stifling of tears and modulation of laughter are just two prominent symptoms of our arrhythmicity.

There are other symptoms: an obsessional feeling one always has to be on schedule, an inability to let emotional experiences take their course, an inability to truly enjoy relationships and events that are not task-oriented, a refusal to admit when strong feelings interfere with the desire or capacity to continue what one is doing, difficulty coping with illness (one's own and those of others), an inability to rest and take time to heal, and so forth.

To the extent we suffer from pathological arrhythmicity we try to avoid all manner of cycles: dependence and independence; happiness and sadness; good fortune and bad; illness and health; potency and impotence. For instance, in an intimate relationship each partner will occasionally be dependent on the other, in what one hopes is some kind of reciprocal alternating rhythm. When the man is unable to tolerate thinking of himself as dependent, he tries to make it appear as if his partner is the dependent one. (Ironically, it is possible to depend on being depended on.) And men who are least tolerant of cycles in themselves tend to devalue most the cyclical experiences of women— hence the male insensitivity to PMS.

A degree of arrhythmicity that is functional at the work place can be constricting in the personal realm. For instance, it can interfere with the capacity to be intimate or to be fully relaxed and playful. When priorities shift and a man who has been steady enough to reach a certain stature in the world of work begins to realize what he has been missing, he might enter psychotherapy. In contrast to women who would like to learn to control their cyclic distress, these men at midlife would be happy to jettison steadiness in favor of more spontaneity and playfulness. I will illustrate the point with an exerpt from my journal.

Crash!

Journal Entry 7/26/1977

CRASH!
Wreck. Car totalled! Could have been killed. Gawd!
How scary! Didn't know what hit me. So powerless.
Distracted by random thoughts intruding on my very
efficient schedule. Could have been killed. Wind-

*shield smashed. Couldn't focus. Dazed. Thought it was
all over.*

*How can this thing interfere with my life!; my
growing list of accomplishments. I can't stick around
the crash site. I need to pick up my kids, get to the
airport. File for divorce. Write an article. Make
money. Fuck! What happened to leisure? Being in
touch with myself? I've got every minute scheduled. I
took a thirty minute lunch break today, sat in my
office with the door closed and spaced out—at last,
breathing space. Then ran into a friend in the hall, felt
uptight, no time to talk—but we hadn't seen each
other in months.*

*Why a crash now? I've been running down for
days. Intense weekend. A little depressed Monday.
Cold, low-energy at work. Damn, I can't keep up this
pace. Why am I running so fast? I told a patient that
he's too busy accumulating commodities. A lawyer, for
him commodities are the number of cases he's won,
the money he makes, the fame, the sexual conquests.
Like capitalism, where the rate of profit must
continually accelerate or there's a crash, this man's
midlife crisis occurs when the rate of accumulating
accomplishments levels off—panic! But it's not just
my patient, it's me, too! I do the same.*

*Then I don't want to accept help. Didn't even
want Mary to stick around at the scene (a co-worker
who was driving by when the crash occurred). Wanted
to rent a car and drive on—like in the Indy 500 when
they come in for a pit stop—wanted to get the kids on
time. Don't be late! Don't ask another parent to pick
up your kids for you! A sign of failure. Failed
steadiness. Dropped the pace. What's the matter with
you, you can't keep up with your commitments?*

The entry ends here. I was in the midst of divorce proceedings, I
was getting used to being a part-time father, and I was trying to further
my career. I felt too small for the monumental tasks I was being asked
to perform. I hoped that by speeding up a little and maintaining a
slightly quicker pace I could pull my life together. I would soon learn,
while undergoing intensive psychotherapy, that by quickening my
pace I was numbing myself to all the very intense feelings that would
otherwise accompany the events of my life.

It is as if we men are running over a large grate in the road, perpendicular to the bars, the spaces between bars being exactly the length of our stride, so that if we were to slow down we would fall between the bars. The problem is that the speed required keeps increasing, so we have to figure out ways to increase our efficiency and stay apace. As we are racing along we keep getting distracted by things we see and hear, but focusing on them causes us to slow the pace and risk slipping between the bars. This is especially true when we pass other people and feel like sharing things we have seen or heard or felt, but know that doing so would cause us to slow our pace and slip.

As we get more tired we begin to believe it would be better to slow down and just let ourselves fall wherever we might, even if into the dark and cold beneath our feet. What frightens us there? The unknown? A dark place? Would we feel our pain? We lose our concentration and begin to stumble. Our bodies are jarred as our feet fall off-center and our joints begin to ache from all the jarring. It is as if we are stumbling, but want it to be always forward, and we keep running merely to make certain our motion will be forward rather than downward, but we no longer care about the pain and the damage to our bodies all the jarring is causing. Finally, when we can not keep it up any longer, we fall between the slats, feeling terror, and not a little relief. Therapists often hear about this kind of relief, but the men who report feeling it consider it to be a symptom of their depression.

Saul

When Saul first entered my consulting room he insisted we talk first about my fee. We arrived at a fee and he relaxed a little. Perhaps he was relieved that I was on his payroll; my financial dependence meant that he did not have to see himself as the only needy one in this encounter. He proceeded to tell me that he would never have been able to talk about these things with the men who share his fast-paced, competitive life. But since he trusted I would be professional and guard his confidentiality, he decided to tell me about personal problems that troubled him.

His wife was the main problem, he explained. She was threatening to leave him because "she's not getting enough out of the relationship." He did not understand. He had never been very emotional or forthcoming with his inner experiences. But he was good to her in other ways. He was a good provider (though she thought his income was not high enough), and he took care of their children evenings and weekends.

"But I've always kept to myself in terms of feelings. When I'm depressed, I just want to be alone, to curl up in bed and blank out the whole world—including her. But I've always been like that. Why is she so upset about it now?"

He told me of coming into the kitchen from the yard where he had been working on the sprinkler system one Sunday. His wife told him she would like to talk to him. He was impatient and told her to get right to the point. Flustered, she became inarticulate. She said she did not really have a particular point, it was more a feeling, she just wanted to talk. He turned and stamped out of the house to finish his project so he could turn the water back on in the house before dark. She spent her next therapy session telling her therapist that this kitchen encounter left her feeling very sad, but she concluded it was her fault for being so inarticulate, so "needy and hysterical." Saul told me that he also felt bad about the encounter. He had felt torn, wanting to be responsive to his wife but also needing to keep moving if he was to finish his project before dark. He also admitted that he felt good when his wife was able to express a need succinctly and he was able to satisfy it, but when

"she's just being needy and wanting to keep me around, and there's really nothing I can do to make her feel better, I feel dragged down into her depression."

The urgency of the job in the garden saved him from having to be near his wife while both experienced uncomfortable feelings, and he was unwilling to let such feelings slow his pace.

Asked to explain his need to withdraw and be alone, he said he always felt a need to hide his "weak spots," something he was taught to do when he was a child. No one wanted to hear about his feelings. His father told him men should not cry. Once while his father was coaching his little league team, Saul was hit in the face with a baseball. His father shook him and told him to stop crying and get back to his position:

"What's the matter, do you want the other kids to think you're a sissy?"

His mother was no more interested in his feelings—in fact she was chronically depressed and incapable of responding to him with empathy. Then there were the schoolmates who laughed at him when he cried after another boy hit him in a fight. Saul learned early to restrain any display of emotion and vulnerability.

"That's the image that got me where I am today. Now she says it's not good enough, there's something wrong with me because I'm not capable of telling her every little detail that's on my mind and everything I feel."

Several months into his therapy Saul contracted a case of the flu and had to stay home. The longer he was home, the more depressed and withdrawn he became. He canceled a session because he was not feeling well enough to come to my office. The next day he called to see if we might reschedule. He seemed agitated when he arrived at the make-up session, and reported a nightmare wherein he was beaten up by another man and humiliated in front of a crowd of onlookers. He wondered whether the dream represented his ongoing rivalry with a co-worker, a man whom he described as "your all-American boy." This other man had been a star athlete and student body president in high school, went to the "right" college, and knew how to "pal around with the old boys" who ran the corporation where they both worked. He, on the other hand, had felt awkward and unpopular in high school and college and still felt uncomfortable at office cocktail parties. The two men were currently vying for a promotion, and while he was home in bed Saul worried that his illness might cause him to fall behind in the race for that promotion.

Among the onlookers in the nightmare was a woman who he said looked a little like a girl he would have liked to date in high school, but who was dating an older guy, "a jock." Until this point in the session, he had been sitting in a slumped position looking at the floor. He looked up and asked if I thought that girl might not also be his wife, and if perhaps his reluctance to share his feelings with her was related to the shame he felt about not being "the all-American boy."

This association led us to a discussion of dependency in his marriage. He told me that until recently he had felt that his wife was very dependent on him, "clingy, as a matter of fact." Recently she had been very successful in a business venture and had established a circle of successful women friends who helped to boost her confidence. She seemed to rely on him less while demanding more of him in the way of emotional forthrightness.

"I guess she is getting support from her women friends and doesn't need me as much any more. That's why she is more critical. I kind of miss her clinginess—I used to enjoy her needing to be with me all the time—as long as there was something I could do to help her with her problems. Now she prefers to be with her friends."

He recalled that he enjoyed his mother's company most when she was depressed, but only if there was something he could do to cheer her up. He never felt that she wanted to hear about his feelings, but knowing she needed him was always reassuring.

Saul's is a classic case of pathological arrhythmicity. He was not able to express his emotions because doing so would amount to a break in the steadiness he congratulated himself on maintaining. Not surprisingly, he did not know his true desires, he spent so much time meeting the requirements of success that he had lost sight of what he really wanted. He had been attracted to his wife because she seemed so vital, but a vital woman craves emotional contact and eventually tires of relating to a man who cannot provide it.

The Man's Dilemma

Men dread natural rhythms, as if cycles threaten the time-and-motion efficiency of working life. But there are deeper, less conscious reasons for our dread. As I pointed out in Chapter One, in a male world there are only two positions, topdog and fallen subordinate. If a man wants to avoid missing a step and falling into a subordinate position, he must learn to function smoothly, efficiently, and regularly. There is no time to take off when one is serious about one's work or one's projects. There is no time to pay attention to the inner life. Besides, there is really no one to talk to about personal matters—other men cannot be trusted because they are just as intent on getting ahead by climbing over others. (Women, too, are perfectly capable of climbing over others, even though one hopes that with more women entering public life there might be less competition and more cooperation.) So one learns to cover up, to hide one's pains and depressions, and to get the job done without divulging anything about one's inner self.

Some men attribute all the tensions in a primary relationship to the woman's emotional dyscontrol. They say she is hysterical, or at least "on the rag." Men are very even-keeled and hope for the same kind of steadiness from partners. But the man's obsession with steadiness causes problems in intimate relationships. After all, quality intimacy is more cyclical than steady. There is a lengthening and shortening of the distance between partners, moments when one is more dependent on the other and others when the roles are reversed, there are intermittent battles followed by resolutions, and then there are more battles.

Two recent movies, *Regarding Henry* and *The Doctor*, offer interesting commentaries on the successful male's steady pace and avoidance of dark, uncertain places within. As *Regarding Henry* opens, Harrison Ford as Henry is a cocky, fast-paced attorney who does not have time to feel connected to colleagues or family. In *The Doctor*, William Hurt as Dr. Jack McGhee moves from operating room to operating room making jokes that are thinly veiled sadistic attacks on patients who are burdened by human frailties such as fear of disfigurement or death. Then something happens. Henry is shot in the head and suffers brain damage, Dr. McGhee discovers he has cancer. There is a transformation. Both men slow down, become more human and vulnerable, develop more sympathy for people who suffer, and learn to value their connectedness with other human beings.

Next, as a more sensitive person, both of these men run into difficulty in the professional worlds they once ruled. Henry discovers that, as a fast-paced attorney, he had lied to win cases, and Jack discovers that a partner of his had tampered with medical charts in order to reduce his liability in a malpractice case—and expects Jack to vouch for the veracity of the altered charts. Both men refuse to play the game any longer. Henry turns the evidence over to the opposing side and Jack refuses to make good his pre-cancer promise to back up the partner. Henry leaves the practice of law. Jack continues as a surgeon after his cancer is cured, but practices very differently, for instance ordering the residents he is training to spend time role-playing as patients in the hospital so that in the future they will be able to empathize with the patients on whom they operate.

A patient in therapy tells me of seeing both movies and then having a dream. He is the manager of a large enterprise, and is very competent at work. But as a person, he is rather closed and unable to share his feelings, even with his wife. He dreams he is driving past a group of people who are doing something secretively. They look at him menacingly, as if they do not want him to pay too close attention to what they are doing. He drives on. The dream's interpretation is obvious to him: At work he often finds himself looking away, ignoring the human side of his encounters so that he can manage effectively. For instance, he had to fire an underling recently, in spite of the fact that the man has three children and little likelihood, given the economy, of finding another job. He identified with both Henry and Jack McGhee, and admits that he is afraid he will meet a tragic end. He wonders whether he hides his feelings so that nobody will know how anxious he is about his own mortality.

Men worry lest too much empathy with a woman's emotional experience will lead to the realization that men can be totally compelled by intense feelings, too. Men pathologize women's natural experiences—menses, pregnancy, menopause—because they do not want to admit that they too might periodically be overcome by bodily experiences and transiently incapable of carrying on with regular responsibilities. In other words, men project onto women the attributes they cannot tolerate in themselves, and then they pathologize those qualities in women.

Jean Baker Miller (1976) comments:

> Once a group is defined as inferior, the superiors tend to label it as defective or substandard in various ways. These labels accrete rapidly. Thus, blacks are described as less intelligent than whites, women are supposed to be ruled by emotion, and so on.... Inevitably, the dominant group is the model for "normal human relationships." (pp. 6–8)

This certainly helps explain why men so readily diagnose PMS in women who periodically become emotional and unsteady.

We should not limit this discussion to menstrual cycles. There is also the cycle of life and death. Sylvia Perara (1981), among others, links the woman's psychological development to the cycles that characterize her life. Perara tells the story of Innana, the Sumerian Goddess of Heaven and Earth, who decides one day to go into the Underworld. She descends, instructing her friend that if she does not return in three days the friend should appeal to the gods to intervene with Ereshkigal, Goddess of the Underworld, to arrange for her return.

When Innana descends, Ereshkigal is furious about the intrusion, kills her, and hangs her body on a post. When Innana does not return, the god Enki intervenes and secures her release. However, Innana must arrange for a substitute to descend to the Underworld in her place (compare the Greek myth of Persephone). Perera comments on the Sumerian myth: "This myth shows us how those dark, repressed levels may be raised, and how they may enter conscious life—through emotional upheavals and grief—to radically change conscious energy patterns" (p. 15). Men, if they can avoid pathologizing the woman's experience, might learn from women that a willingness to fully experience descents into darkness is a prerequisite to transforming one's life.

Saying that men have much to learn from women is not the same as saying that the ways of women are better than the ways of men. The point is that male and female ways have become polarized, to the detriment of both genders, and the male proclivity to pathologize women's experience merely causes further polarization. Consider the difference between men and women in regard to the timing of sexual desire. Many marital storms begin because the man does not feel the woman is interested in sex frequently or regularly enough, while he likes regular sexual contact and depends on it to bolster his confidence in his manliness. This is not a case where the man's or the woman's sexual cravings are more natural or correct. In fact, in terms of the survival of the species, there must have been times when men's and women's contrasting sexual rhythms worked in harmony. Since ovulation occurs in monthly cycles, men's readiness to engage in sexual intercourse at any time of the month maximizes the liklihood of fertilization, the man being ready whenever the woman happens to be ovulating and receptive. For the modern couple the exigencies of natural selection are not as important and there are layers of cultural and psychological issues superimposed over the biological substrate. The challenge for couples is to work out a sexual timetable that takes into account the cyclic desires of the woman as well as the steadier urges of the man, does not involve coercion or guilt, and results in an adequate degree of mutual satisfaction.

Helmut Barz (1991) challenges the idea that, if men could just become more like women, the world would be a better place. He explains that even if a man is totally in touch with his feminine side and a woman with her masculine side, the two sexes would still be quite different, and the goal of self-realization for men and women should not be a unisex ideal. As if discussing the roots of pathological arryhthmicity in men, Barz writes: "When the exclusively masculine spirit loses the feminine form of the spirit, whose strength lies in the capacity for lovingly related syntheses, it degenerates into a dissecting tool—powerfully masculine, to be sure, but ultimately destructive of life" (p. 28).

There is a link between the tendency in men to ignore their own natural rhythms (nature within), and a proclivity to destroy the environment (nature outside). There is the same attempt to override nature, and in both cases the overriding is combined with the incessant drive to beat the competition in order to amass status, power, and wealth. I have discussed men's need to override their natural cycles in order to maintain a steady pace so they can be competitive at work and climb higher in the hierarchy. In regard to the environment, the men who direct large industrial enterprises claim there is simply not enough time, and the costs would be prohibitive, to slow production and figure out a way to preserve the ozone layer and the rainforests.

The Persian Gulf War presented many examples of pathological arrhythmicity. President Bush did not even miss a stroke when, in the middle of a round of golf, he received news of Iraq's invasion of Kuwait and ordered American troops to the region. Then, after ordering more than 400,000 troops to Saudi Arabia, he gave Americans a rationale for war that they could finally understand: Real men do not back down. Saddam Hussein repeatedly matched Bush's call for men to act as real men, for instance in his accusation that American forces demonstrated cowardice by pursuing a prolonged air assault and avoiding the more manly pastime of ground warfare. The message from both leaders betrays severe pathological arrhythmicity. In this social climate, is it any wonder that the natural rhythms of women are pathologized while men's inhuman arrhythmicity is not?

The Social Construction of Gender

In my view, biology does not determine gender relations; gender is socially constructed. Of course, biology matters. The males and females of all species have different roles, if only because females bear children. But just about everything else about human gender relations is shaped by culture in its historical permutations. (For a review of the debate between "biological determinists" and "social constructivists," see Kessler and McKenna, 1978; for a critique of "biological determinism," see Schifellite, 1987.)

Notice that I am arguing both that gender is socially constructed and that problems result when men override their "natural" cycles. Is there a contradiction between these two arguments? I think not. Human beings are not ruled by "natural" cycles. We interpret nature around and within us in relation to our social/cultural context. But each gender, in a particular social/cultural context, adopts a stance in relation to natural cycles. Women are not biologically fated to maintain natural rhythms for the collectivity. Men can serve that function as well; consider the sun dance of American Plains Indians wherein men pierce their chests so that their blood will spill on the ground, symbolizing the (male) sun's importance in the fertility of mother earth. I am arguing that women and men alike are all too willing to connect themselves to the tempo of a competitive marketplace and public life, a tempo that upsets natural rhythms in a particular, gendered way. If one is to understand the arrhythmicity of men, it is important to understand why the rhythms of women are pathologized.

The advance of civilization, particularly since the Industrial Revolution, has made us slaves to the clock (Mumford, 1934). Where agricultural societies regulated activities according to natural rhythms—the rising and setting of the sun, the seasons of the year—with the advent of modern technology and factory organization, the clock has replaced the sun and the moon as the measure of time. The worker's activities, from the rate of productivity to the frequency of visits to the bathroom, is regulated by the clock (Thompson, 1967).

Service and white collar workers are no better off: the number of cases or clients can be measured, as can the bulk of paperwork.

With time and work thus quantified, people learn to do things they might once have considered unnatural. They wake with alarms, work nights, and wear out their bodies doing monotonous tasks. Men appear to have adapted well to such demands, and many women have also proven quite skilled as they rise to places of prominence previously reserved for men only. But women have to pay a high price for their entry into the top echelons of a previously all male world. They, too, are becoming alienated from nature; for instance, they must learn not to let their premenstrual symptoms or their plans to have children interfere with their reliability on the job.

Does the fact that women experience certain discomfiting states just prior to menses necessarily mean they suffer from a mental disorder; that the problem is internal to the woman? Perhaps the woman's problem, as well as the man's, does not lie with the woman's psychopathology, but rather with a disorder in our very "civilized" relationship to nature and to natural rhythms. Premenstrual sadness might be understood as a period of mourning for a missed opportunity to bear a child, a moment to pause, to grieve, perhaps to take a deep breath before reentering the bustling outside world. Many cultures have rituals to mark and honor this time in the woman's cycle. In the complicated modern world of work, the menstrual cycle becomes something else. The premenstrual woman today is less likely concerned about rituals; less likely to measure time by the cycles of the moon; and more likely to curse the fact that she is a month older, that her body holds her back, or that she has not been as successful as she had hoped to be by this time in her life. Where once the cycles of a woman's body seemed to fit the rhythms of a culture, today the woman's monthly changes in body and mood are not well tolerated in the male workplace—and the lack of tolerance can turn transient mournful sadness into depression and self-castigation.

A working woman is told she must ignore her natural rhythms if she is to fit into a man's world and excel. The woman must learn to endure, just like a man. If, at times in her cycle, she feels bodily pain, she can take medications to increase her tolerance. If the pains are emotional and spiritual, then she may find psychotherapy helpful, or turn to psychotropic medications. Using whatever help she can get, the woman, if she wants to play by the rules and succeed, must prove the sexist assumptions of her boss wrong and demonstrate that she can be as steady and reliable as any man.

This is a big source of tension for many women. A female executive recently complained:

"I feel trapped, if I play their (male) game they promote me, but I become one of them; if I don't play I don't get the promotion; either way, I lose."

Schwartz (1989) suggests that women, if they want to have a career and a family, be placed on a "Mommy track" at work, a slower track that delays career advancement and limits ultimate achievement but permits time off for the woman to raise children. Diane Ehrensaft (1990) points out that men have always had children and not had to sacrifice their status in the world of work: "Translation: If you're a woman who wants to make it to the top, forget children; if you're a corporate man who wants to be a father, no problem" (p. 63).

Will the influx of women in record numbers into the work force and the ranks of managers and professionals serve to diminish arrhythmicity, the use of intimidation by those who wield power, cutthroat competition, and insensitivity to personal feelings? Of course, the answer depends on whether women change themselves in order to fit in or insist that workplace relations change. There are women in positions of power who try very hard to be as aggressive, competitive, and emotionally closed as men. Then there is the San Jose policewoman who was interviewed on television news recently saying she is not as large as a man and speaks in a "squeaky voice" instead of a "loud roar," so she does not intimidate anyone when she arrives on a scene and must find other ways to calm a situation down. The conclusion one draws from the news segment is that policewomen find ways to negotiate settlements in situations where policemen typically resort to intimidation and force. The presence of a large number of women at work and in public life who would like to find alternatives to intimidation and cutthroat competition could lead to big changes in the way business and public life are conducted.

Meanwhile men in record numbers are visiting therapists, joining groups, and gathering at large men's meetings and conferences in order to find a way to break through the arrhythmicity that erodes the possibility of change and drains their vitality. Of course, they do not understand their symptoms in terms of pathological arrhythmicity, but when I point out to the men who come to my consulting room the connection between their sense of inner deadness, their troubled intimacies, and the requirement that they maintain a steady pace in order to succeed at work, they quickly get the point. It takes courage for men to cross the lines that delineate traditional manly virtues. And it takes courage for men to admit that their arryhthmicity causes as many problems as does women's PMS.

CHAPTER THREE

Homophobia in Straight Men

Afew years ago I toured a high-security prison in the Midwest as an expert witness in litigation concerning the effects of prison conditions on prisoners' mental health. When I stepped into the main entry area of the prison, I saw a woman milling around with the men a short distance down one of the halls. She was blond, slim, very feminine—or so I thought on first glance. Actually, "she" was a young man, perhaps 21, dressed as a woman. Blond, blue-eyed, slight and sensuous, he played the part very well. He wore a flowing red gown that reached the floor, had a shawl draped across his chest in a way that did not permit one to assess the size of his breasts, wore make-up, and sported a very seductive female pose. I was surprised to see an attractive woman roaming around in a men's prison. One of the attorneys accompanying me on the tour told me with a wink that "she" was a he, and asked if I would like to talk to him.

The inmate told me he was not really gay, and certainly did not believe he would dress as a woman again after he was released, but on "the inside" it's the only way for him to survive unless he "locks up"; that is, asks for protective custody in a segregated section of the prison where inmates who do not feel safe on the "mainline" are housed, including those identified as "snitches" and child molesters. When this man arrived at the prison at 19 he was beat up and raped a number of times, and on several other occasions prison toughs fought with each other for the opportunity to use him sexually. He learned that it was safer to become the "woman" of a tough prisoner, that way he would not be beaten nor be the object of rivalries between prison toughs. He would become the passive sexual partner of one dominant man.

Later that day I met with a group of security officers. One mentioned the young man. I said I had met him. The officer asked if I'd like to hear the bit of advice he would have given that slight and fair young man if he had seen him when he entered the prison. Before I had a chance to answer, he blurted out:

"What you want to do is the first time you go out on the yard you break off a metal bed post and shove it down your trouser leg. Then, when a big guy comes up and pinches your ass or makes a lewd remark, you pull out the metal stick and smack him as hard as you can across the face. You'll both get thrown in the hole for ten days. Then, when you get out, everyone will respect you as a 'crazy' and no one will hassle you for sex any more."

In prison, "butt-fucking" is the symbol of dominance. The strong do it, the weak must submit. Homosexual rape is a constant threat for those who cannot prove they are "man enough." According to Tom Cahill (1990), a survivor of prison rape: "We are victims of a system in which those who are dominated and humiliated come to dominate and humiliate others" (p. 33). Perhaps this explains why prisoners do so much body-building.

Free men do a lot of toughening, too. If it is not the physique it's the mind, or it's the reputation or the financial empire, but men are always building something that they believe will keep them off the bottom of the heap, out of range of those who would "shaft" them. This is not a complete explanation of men's competitiveness and defensiveness—competition is built into our social relations—but men's subjective dread of "being shafted" plays a part in sustaining those competitive social relations. The prison drama reverberates in the male psyche. It is as if men do not want to appear incapable of defending themselves against rape at any time. We stiffen our bodies when approached by other men who want to touch or hug and we keep men at a certain distance—where we can watch them and be certain that closeness and dependency will not make us too vulnerable.

Homophobia in Everyday Life

Weinberg (1972) defines homophobia: "The dread of being in close quarters with homosexuals." Pharr (1988) defines it as: "Societal hatred, rejection, or fear of gay and lesbian people." According to Cabaj (1985), the definition should also include hatred of the idea of homosexuality, hatred of the expression of affection between two members of the same sex, the motivation behind attacks on gays ("gay-bashing"), and a form of self-hatred among gay people. Weeks (1981) and Duroche (1991) uncover the roots of homophobia in the nineteenth century when "deep male bonding began to be perceived as a threat, to the individual as well as to the social order" (Duroche, 1991, p. 3). Morin and Garfinkle (1978a) studied the personality correlates of homophobia in men and concluded that they tend to be authoritarian, rigid, intolerant of ambiguity, concerned about status, conflicted about their sexual impulses, and distancing with others. Malyon (1982) discusses "internalized homophobia" in gay men, but I will restrict this discussion to homophobia in straight men.

Homophobia is about fear and hatred of gays and lesbians, it is also about the stiffening and the distancing men do with other men, regardless of sexual orientation. Straight men fear close contact with each other and try to avoid doing anything that others might interpret as effeminate or unmanly. Homophobia can be subtle and unconscious. Fantasies as primitive as being "butt-fucked" usually remain unconscious until men explore their homophobia and discover the fantasies that lurk behind their fears. It is the subtle and unconscious forms of homophobia that constrict the lives and possibilities of sensitive heterosexual men.

Men do not enter my consulting room asking if I can help them overcome their homophobia. And most of the men I treat would never knowingly discriminate against gays and lesbians. Their homophobia is much more subtle. For instance, a male client speaks disparagingly about a gay colleague. I ask what the other man represents to him. He assures me he would never support any kind of discrimination against gays in the workplace. Next he recalls his father jeering at him whenever he did not seem to be trying hard enough in sports to suit the older man: "What's the matter, are you queer?" He realizes that the thing that bothers him most about his gay colleague is his lack of athletic prowess: "It's not so much that he's effeminate, though he is that, but he's so flabby and uncoordinated, he looks like he's never thrown a ball or run a race." This client lifts weights daily and very consciously keeps his chest out and his stomach in at all times. He quickly sees the connection between this discussion—a discussion about homophobia even though we never use the term—and a complaint that was on his original list of reasons for seeking psychotherapy, his concern that he is "wound up tighter than the spring on a clothespin." And he originally wanted me to help him "relax and be more playful."

Men tell me they would like to have close male friends, then they add they do not want me to get the idea they are gay. In other words, homophobia plays a part in their isolation and inability to sustain meaningful same-sex intimacies. Other men want to quit coming to see me as soon as the symptoms that motivated them to seek therapy diminish a little. When we explore the reasons they might want to terminate so abruptly, we discover their fear of becoming dependent on another man, or their fear of the affection that is developing between us. Of course, their fears are not entirely a matter of homophobia. They have had very real experiences of betrayal and abuse at the hands of men upon whom they were once dependent, beginning with their fathers. But homophobia is a relevant issue.

On several occasions when I have confronted male clients about their need to terminate therapy abruptly, we have discovered that they had sexual feelings toward me, or were afraid I had sexual feelings toward them. In cases where the client has been willing to continue in therapy and explore these fantasies, we have reached the conclusion that the wish to flee from psychotherapy is a defense against complicated and conflictual feelings about the expression of affection between two men and its connection to homosexuality. Homophobia is an important part of male psychology, even in men who would never knowingly support any kind of overt discrimination against gays and lesbians.

Al's Dream

Al had been in therapy with me for six months when he reported a dream. At the end of a romantic evening out, including dinner, a jazz club and not a few drinks, he tried to seduce his wife. She politely let him know she was not feeling very sexual, and when he fell asleep he had this dream: A group of escaped prisoners have broken into his house and taken him and his wife captive. He is stripped, bent over, and repeatedly raped. Then his wife is stripped and forced to the floor next to him. He is made to watch as the largest intruder commences to rape her.

Al is frightened by the dream, but also reports he felt excited when he waked. We discuss its meaning. There is the prisoner who rapes his wife, expressing the rage he sometimes feels toward her, and perhaps the man's size reflects Al's belief that if he were "more of a man" she would be more "turned on" by him. The image of his wife being compelled to have sex puts him in touch with his wish to compel her, as well as the wish that she would be the one to compel him to have sex sometimes. And he tells me, with some embarrassment, that anal rape may represent the defeat and humiliation he feels every time his wife refuses his advances—he admits he often wonders if she might be having an affair while using her tiredness as a way to hide it from him. He begins to see the link between his feelings of inadequacy and his fear that weak men are at risk of rape at the hands of more dominant men.

It is not easy for Al to examine his unconscious associations to this dream, he is horrified that he is capable of imagining such bestiality. Every image and feeling contradicts his view of himself as a strong, sensitive man. Meanwhile, he complains of chronic tiredness and lack of interest in anything. Obviously an aim of Al's therapy will be to help him channel some of the dream's aggressive and erotic energy into the areas of his life where currently he feels a lack of passion. But first he must confront his deep feelings of inadequacy, and the concerns he has about his own manliness that get stirred up whenever his wife refuses his advances.

On Being Turned Into a Woman

Plenty of very homophobic men vicariously enjoy the explicit depiction of sex between women in pornographic magazines and videos. Seeing two women involved in sexual acts is not threatening, perhaps because one can fantasize entering both women. What the homophobic man fears is not sex between people of the same gender, but rather passive sex, wherein the male is penetrated anally. A man can respect a woman, protect her from abuse by others, and appreciate her femaleness, but to be *like her* is a totally revolting thought, especially in regard to penetration by a man. John Ross (1986) links men's fears of intimacy with women as well as their ambivalence about fatherhood with an underlying dread of being turned into a woman.

Men insult each other in telling ways—"You have no balls," "You cry like a woman," "Don't be a w-o-o-s-s," "What a pussy"—in other words, the worst thing a man can call another is a woman. Men remember the schoolyard scenario where the guy who wins the fight is lauded while the guy who "chickens out" or gets "his ass whipped" is devalued, the worst humiliation being when others call him a girl. This is why the prison scenario reverberates with such intensity in the male psyche. Jean Genet (1966) reports that he learned how to be a prison tough while still at Mettray reform school: "Bulkaen, on the other hand, was a little man whom Mettray had turned into a girl for the use of the big shots, and all his gestures were the sign of nostalgia for his plundered, destroyed virility" (p. 144).

Forstein (1988) locates the problem of homophobia in the need on the part of straight men to compensate for their insecurities: "Those who are truly heterosexually oriented, but insecure and uncomfortable with the orientation and the implied role, may exaggerate what they perceive to be evidence that they are indeed heterosexual. These individuals may manifest homophobic attitudes in an attempt to confirm their heterosexuality to themselves and others" (p. 34).

Peggy Reeves Sanday's (1990) study of fraternity gang rape uncovers blatant homophobia among the fraternity members who participate. Coeds who are insecure about their popularity are invited to the frat house, plied with drinks and drugs, and then seduced by a fraternity brother. Other brothers, who may have been watching the initial sexual encounter, then enter the room and proceed to have serial sex with the coed, who is too inebriated to know what is happening, much less to protest. Sanday interviews fraternity members at two different universities who have participated in what they call "pulling train," and found that most believe the women gave their implicit consent by being at the frat house and accepting the booze and drugs, and these young men do not think they have done anything wrong. Sanday comments:

> Men entice one another into the act of "pulling train" by implying that those who do not participate are unmanly or homosexual. This behavior is full of contradictions because the homoeroticism of "pulling train" seems obvious. A group of men watch each other having sex with a woman who may be unconscious. One might well ask why the woman is even necessary for the sexual acts these men stage for one another. As fraternity practices described in this book suggest, the answer seems to lie in homophobia. One can suggest that in the act of "pulling train" the polymorphous sexuality of homophobic men is given a strictly heterosexual form. (p. 12)

When a man considers wearing a colorful or flamboyant article of clothing, has the impulse to hug or kiss another man in public, toys with the idea of donning an unusual hair style, or wants to take a ballet class—all things women do with abandon—he must consider what others will think. Will they think I am too effeminate? Maybe they will think I am gay. The thought stops us. Here is another of those lines a man is not supposed to cross. Weinberg (1972) includes in his list of reasons for men's homophobia the repressed envy straight men feel toward gays because of the freedom ascribed to gays. In other words, straight men despise homosexuals because they envy gay men's freedom from traditional gender roles. Few men admit they feel this kind of envy, but I believe it plays a part in homophobia. A male client tells me his wife is developing a close friendship with a gay man:

"I don't mind, really. I'm not jealous or anything. It's just that, when they spend time together they laugh and get silly, then they cry together about another friend who's got AIDS, and they just seem to get into this emotional space with each other. She and I haven't had that kind of emotional contact in years. I envy his ability to get into that space with her. I guess I am a little jealous."

But envy is not the most significant reason for homophobia.

In the heterosexual male imagination, the thought of homosexuality is closely associated with the threat of violence—involuntary sodomy by a more powerful male. The link is usually unconscious, but not very far beneath the surface. Of course, if a straight man does not wish to be penetrated anally, the only way it can happen is violently—and no "real man" would ever let that occur without putting up a ferocious fight. Fantasies of domination and submission are enacted with particular fury in prison. Men watching Tom Selleck play a falsely imprisoned middle class man who murders a tough black inmate in An Innocent Man are very ready to believe that a man is justified in committing murder to avoid anal rape. When straight men think of being penetrated, they think of violence. There is no other way.

The inability to acknowledge any homosexual impulses in oneself causes men to project all homosexual desires outward, onto gay men. Since the only way a straight man can conceive of having sex with a man is rape, and since gay men are the only ones who have an urge to make love with another man, the anxious straight concludes that only a gay man would be a threat. Thus the gay-basher aims to beat up or kill gay men in order to lessen the likelihood he will ever be forced to engage in sex with a man. On this issue Freud was correct, one can protest too much, latent homosexuality is at the core of homophobia. Freud erred only when his own homophobia led him to pathologize homosexuality.

Outside of prison, the fear of anal rape is linked to men's obsession with the question who is on top, the man dreading the loss of a battle and the fall to the bottom of the heap. Boys are taught the link between homosexuality and violence on the schoolyard, where "weakling," "loser," "chicken," "girl," and "queer" are all synonymous. The link lasts for life. We always stand ready to fight like a man. Of course, most men move on from the fist fights of the schoolyard to more adult forms of competition, be that a ferocious legal battle, a romantic rivalry or an effort to beat the competition and clinch the deal or the promotion. Men's fantasies do not entirely explain competition, but in a society where competition is the name of the game they serve to motivate men to continue competing. In the straight male imagination, anal rape is the penalty for losing and being dominated. The imagined disgrace intensifies the drive to move upward in every hierarchy.

The presence of gay men is a constant reminder to anxious straights that "butt-fucking" remains a possibility. Just as rape is more an expression of violent hatred against women than it is a form of sexual desire, homophobia is more about the dread of being violently thrown to the bottom of the heap and disgraced then it is about sexual preference. Homosexuality is not really about rape and violence, it is about desire, eroticism, tenderness and affection between men. The exception is a segment of the gay community where the hypermasculine image reigns, but even here the AIDS epidemic and the need for the gay community to take care of its ill members is causing big changes.

Jeff Beane (1990) writes: "As we continue to evolve and redefine positive identities as gay and bi men, we are freeing ourselves from the restrictive and dysfunctional aspects of male gender role training" (p. 161). Meanwhile the homophobe (and the homophobic part of every man, no matter how subtle and well-contained), intent on denying his craving for affection from other men, projects the sexual desire as well as the violent impulses. Gays are the most available objects of scorn, and there is the added advantage that, in hating gays, the homophobe proves he is not guilty of excessive fondness for men.

Psychotherapy and Homophobia

Psychotherapists are not immune to homophobia, and when they are unaware of their own homophobia it can cause them to be biased in their treatment of men who are conflicted about their gender identity and sexual preference. James Coleman (1973) writes about his disappointment in the two therapists he saw over a span of several years. Both denied they were biased about homosexuality, but then proved otherwise when he talked about his conflicts:

> Twice while in therapy, I met homosexual acquaintances with whom the possibility of a real relationship existed, and shunned them. A therapist might usefully have explored why I was so guilty, even urged me to overcome this guilt; instead, these occurrences became evidence that I did not really want to be homosexual (which we already knew) and since my not wanting to be gay was implicitly a sign (perhaps my only sign) of health, these occurrences were not examined critically. Similarly, my therapists

spent much time trying to discover why my relationships with straight friends were so passionate—rather than asking me why I formed these passionate relationships with straights. Similarly, after the homosexual affair which lost me my teaching job—a very warm relationship which continues, intermittently, to this day—I brought to my next therapist the datum that while in bed with my lover, I felt completely harmonious and "natural," not "sick" at all and not even guilty. Although this contradicted the very basis of the feeling which led me to psychotherapy, my therapist never took the initiative in exploring this contradiction. (pp. 500–501)

If Coleman's report is accurate, his therapists are not trying to help him work through his inner conflicts so that he can uncover his deepest desires regarding sexual preference, but rather are trying to impose their own moral stance, a stance grounded in unconscious homophobia. These therapists, while claiming to have no biases, selectively attempt to help him work through the blocks he encounters in heterosexual relationships while offering no help in his attempts to make homosexual relationships work. Even if Coleman's therapists are not fairly described, his description does capture a familiar moment experienced by other clients with other therapists (Morin & Garfinkel, 1978b).

Even though the American Psychiatric Association was forced by gay and lesbian critics to remove homosexuality from the official list of categories of mental illness in 1973, traditional psychoanalysts and psychotherapists continue to pathologize homosexuality. For instance, Reuben Fine (1988) believes that a certain degree of bisexuality is normal and can lead to homosexual experimentation during adolescence, but when overt homosexual behavior continues into adulthood it is a sign of significant emotional disturbance, usually reflecting overinvolvement with a seductive and castrating mother. Basing their interventions on this formulation, traditional therapists focus selectively on the neurotic conflicts that underlie homosexual object choice and ignore the homophobia that constricts men's options and stifles their passion. Can a male client really explore his full range of options with a therapist who is this biased about what constitutes "normal" male inclinations? The psychoanalytic establishment's approach to homosexuality has been criticized for its homophobic biases and lack of social and historical perspective (Bayer, 1981; Marmor, 1980; Murphy, 1984; Friedman, 1986).

Alfred Adler's (1912) theory of "masculine protest" helps us understand the psychological roots of homophobia. According to Adler, the child develops a sense of inferiority because of his or her "familial organic constitution." A twitch, left-handedness, incoordination, weakness, deafness or bed-wetting—depending on how the child's "organ inferiority" is handled in the family—might develop, in the neurotic, "into a deeply-felt sense of inferiority." The neurotic-to-be both accepts passively the family's attribution of inferiority and actively rebels against the attribution, developing a compensatory striving toward power and domination—"the masculine protest." "The neurotic's worldly projects are doomed to continually reenact the drama of a struggle between the masculine (powerful) and feminine (weak, inferior) parts of the psyche, at the expense of real creativity and happiness." Adler did not mention homophobia, but he certainly described its psychological roots.

By 1927 Adler had integrated this psychological formulation with a social analysis:

> All our institutions, our traditional attitudes, our laws, our morals, our customs, give evidence of the fact that they are determined and maintained by privileged males for the glory of male domination. It is very difficult to make it clear to a child that a mother who is engaged in household duties is as valuable as a father. (Adler, 1927, cited in Miller, 1973, p. 40)

Is it any wonder that Freud and Adler parted ways in 1912, mostly because Adler would not accept Freud's phallocentric theories? Still, Adler's concept of "masculine protest" is echoed in the work of other psychoanalyts, for instance, F. Boehm's (1932) idea that hypermasculinity is a defense against a man's unconscious female identification.

Feminists, including Nancy Chodorow (1978), Dorothy Dinnerstein (1976), and Lillian Rubin (1985), further our understanding of homophobia by offering an alternative to the traditional psychoanalytic formulation of the Oedipal phase of development. During that phase the male child "disidentifies" with his mother and begins to relate more to his father (Greenson, 1968). Disidentification does not occur in an instant, the boy deciding he will no longer look or be like his mother in any noticeable regard. Rather, he begins in earnest the process of learning the postures and practices of men, ways to conduct himself more like a man than a woman—a process that will take years and contain many false starts and hairpin turns.

Is it any surprise that many males believe that they must cast aside every feminine trait in order to thoroughly disidentify with mother, for instance no longer permitting their mothers to hug them? After all, boys are taught to think that males do not require very much display of affection—as if clinging to the thought will prevent a boy's missing his mother's arms. It does seem a throwback to this Oedipal dilemma when men, in a burst of insecurity about their masculinity, wonder whether they are too womanly, in other words too much like their mothers. The adult tendency to disidentify strongly with gays has roots in the Oedipal boy's need to disidentify with his mother—the devaluation of women and the expression of hatred toward gays being signs of a "real man."

The search for a strong male identity reappears in force during early adolescence. Boys are especially careful to be unlike girls, even while constantly grooming themselves and eagerly searching for clues to what it is that attracts girls to boys. Boys tend to do cruel things during this period. They humiliate other boys who seem unmanly or "queer," and they devalue girls, for instance, bragging about their sexual conquests. The disidentification is with all females and all feminine traits. Boys are led to believe that if they can only exaggerate the differences between themselves and those men who are willing to be used as women, they can discover the secret to being a man.

It is no accident that Freud pathologized homosexuality as well as womanhood. As Jean Baker Miller (1976) points out, the dominant group always defines the characteristics of subordinate groups as inferior, and in our psychological age, this means the inclinations of subordinate groups are pathologized. Where once psychoanalysts diagnosed penis envy in ambitious women and considered homosexuality a form of mental illness, today's clinicians diagnose late luteal phase dysphoric disorder in women and "psychosexual disorders" in gays and lesbians. The categories change but the potential for gender-bias remains.

Some Social Implications

Homophobia is socially reinforced and solidifies the current social arrangements, including the male theme of topdog and fallen subordinate. Suzanne Pharr (1988) courageously asserts that homophobia is not a peripheral issue in the struggle against sexism—it is not just a matter of protecting the rights of gays and lesbians—rather, homophobia is at the core of sexism and must be routed out if gender relations are to improve significantly. She writes:

> When gay men break ranks with male roles through bonding and affection outside the arenas of war and sports, they are perceived as not being "real men," that is, as being identified with women, the weaker sex that must be dominated and that over the centuries has been the object of male hatred and abuse. Misogyny gets transferred

to gay men with a vengeance and is increased by the fear that their sexual identity and behavior will bring down the entire system of male dominance and compulsory heterosexuality. (p. 19)

Pharr proceeds to examine the role of homophobia in the battering of women.

Homophobia marks a line of demarcation and helps maintain a narrow, traditional definition of masculinity. I often have the urge to put my arm around a male friend's waist as we walk, only to find myself wondering if others will think we are gay. Once I went to a movie with a male friend, and on the way out of the theater saw a male client waiting in line. In the midst of a lively discussion, my friend and I have the habit of touching each other while making points. The client seemed very uncomfortable in our encounter, and called the next day to say he wanted to terminate psychotherapy. Though he denied his decision had anything to do with our meeting at the theater, I was left to wonder whether he had concluded I was gay. I thought about calling him back and asking if my perception was accurate and that he was cutting off contact with me for fear I was gay, but decided against that course of action. What would I have said if he had validated my perception? Of course, I reviewed the incident and tried to decide if I had acted inappropriately, for instance in demonstrating affection toward my friend in public. This is a complicated question for a psychotherapist who comes from a psychoanalytic tradition. I decided I would not act differently in the future; I just do not believe it is inappropriate for men to show their affection toward one another.

I told a gay friend about the incident and he pointed out that while I suffered some discomfort, a gay man who is perceived as gay in the wrong place always has to fear being beaten or killed. As Franklin Abbott (1990) writes about his experience in high school: "If you were ever labelled queer that was it. Your life would be pure hell until you graduated or killed yourself" (p. 232).

There is a homophobic part in every man; socialization is never a total failure. Homophobia is like racism and sexism in this regard. It is impossible to grow up in a culture where homophobia, sexism, and racism are rampant and not internalize a tendency to discriminate to some extent. And the lessons from the struggle to end racism and sexism can be applied in the struggle against homophobia. For instance, W. J. Cash, in The Mind of the South (1941), asks a critical question: Why do poor white Southerners ally with plantation owners in racist organizations like the KKK instead of allying with poor blacks to demand their fair share of the economic pie from the wealthy whites who exploit the poor of both races? Cash concludes that, by allying with plantation owners poor whites are able to identify with their power and thus convince themselves they are not really at the bottom of the heap—at least they are not "niggers." As in the case of the poor white Southerner who joins a racist group, overtly homophobic men are saying:

"I may feel inadequate in many ways, but at least I'm not gay, at least I don't have to bend over and be sodomized by another man."

If one grew up as a white male in this society, remnants of racist, sexist, and homophobic attitudes will remain in the psyche forever. All we can say for certain is that we are men who are trying to rid ourselves of homophobia, just as we are trying to rid ourselves of all vestiges of racism and sexism.

Straights and Gays

Straight men discover it is not easy to associate closely with gays and lesbians; people might get ideas. The problem is exaggerated among straight, image-conscious adolescents, who tend to ostracize gays. A separation of gays and straights occurs, a separation that leads to a lifelong alienation between the groups. The distancing encourages projections, particularly negative ones. This is why some straight men are gullible enough to believe that all gays are pedarasts and should not be permitted to teach young children, or that all gays are alike and actually fit the stereotypes straights have manufactured.

Of course, men who want to move beyond this stereotype must join the struggle to end homophobia in the public arena: the struggle to end discrimination against gays and lesbians at work and in the eyes of the law, to end gay-bashing, to make available adequate resources to fight AIDS, and so forth. This is an important part of the battle against sexism. By keeping straights and gays separate, and by stigmatizing gays, homophobia serves to consolidate the grip of traditional masculinity over the great majority of American men. Homophobia is about the rigidities and closings that are woven into the male psychic structure by a lifetime of admonitions not to be a "weakling," a "loser," a "sissy," or a "queer."

Before the term "homosexual" was invented, Edward Carpenter wrote about "intermediate types," and the possibility they "might fulfill a positive and useful function" (quoted in Thompson, 1987, p. 152). According to Carpenter (1916):

The Uranian (homosexual, gay) temperament in man closely
resembles the normal temperament of women in this respect—that
in both, love, in some form or other, is the main object of life. In
the normal man, ambition, moneymaking, business, adventure, et
cetera, play their part—love is, as a rule, a secondary matter. (cited
in Thompson, 1987, p. 157)

Whether or not Carpenter's generalizations are valid today, he opened
the discussion of a positive social role for gay men. Harry Hay,
"generally acknowledged as the father of gay liberation" (Thompson,
1987, p. 265), founded the Mattachine Society in the early 'fifties and
posed to its gay members three questions: "Who are we gay people?";
"Where have we been throughout the ages?"; and "What might we be
for?"

Many men today are attempting to stop posturing as if they were
warding off penetration at every turn. These men are seeking a third
alternative to the either/or topdog/fallen subordinate schema. But for
the homophobe, and the homophobic part in every straight man, there
is no third alternative. In fact, homophobia is one big reason many
men feel a need to keep fighting their way to the top in every situation.
I believe straight men have much to learn from gays, and vice versa.
Consider the male theme of top and bottom. What is the position of
gay men? To be brutally concrete, when two men make love there is no
assumption that one will be on top and active while the other is on the
bottom and passive, as there is, on the average, when a man and
woman make love. These things remain to be negotiated in each
instance. How are men to negotiate who will be on top? Could the
lessons of sex carry over to the conduct of commerce and politics? Does
someone have to "get shafted" in order for someone else to succeed and
feel good? Straight men have much to learn from gays, if only because
the latter are forced to challenge the reigning gender sensibility if they
are to find a tenable role for themselves in the social drama (Carrigan,
Connell, & Lee, 1987).

Women and gay men have been talking about gender issues for a
long time. They have been forced to, since it is on account of their
gender or their sexual preference that they are oppressed. Straight men
have done much less talking. Of course, it is not the job of women and
gays to show straight men the way to break free. But a free and open
exchange between men and women, straight and gay, would offer a
golden opportunity to examine our gender relations and move forward
together.

CHAPTER FOUR

Men in Couples

I n *The Book of Laughter and Forget-ting*, Milan Kundera (1980) describes a marriage:

> In those first weeks it was decided between Karel and Marketa that Karel would be unfaithful and Marketa would submit, but that Marketa would have the privilege of being the better one in the couple and Karel would always feel guilty. (p. 36)

I do not agree with Kundera that "every love relationship is based on unwritten conventions rashly agreed upon by the lovers during the first weeks of their love" (p. 36). Rather, I believe that the terms of a relationship are always changing, and that only by resolving the tensions that continually creep into the relationship can a couple keep their love alive. But Kundera makes an important point about the unstated ways partners hold their own in the inevitable and ongoing power struggles.

As middle class women enter the world of work in record numbers (less affluent women have always had to work because their families needed two incomes to survive) and men assume shared responsibilities at home there are new sources of relational tensions, including new forms of competition. Who earns more on the job? Who is the better parent? When his turf was the world of work and hers the home, there was less need to compete. Each partner reigned supreme in a different realm. Now, where there is a discrepancy in earning power as well as a discrepancy in domestic competence, and where one or both partners have a need to compete, there are new kinds of envy and rivalry. This is especially true if the discrepancy reflects a reversal of gender roles, the woman earning more and the man doing more than half of the childrearing.

Cary and Sarah married a year after they met in graduate school and have two young children. They are both professionals in their late twenties. He enters individual psychotherapy for depression. He does not know why he is depressed, but the depression drains his energy and he is unable to work. Then, when he comes home he finds he has insufficient energy "to spend quality time with the kids." His wife, he feels, pulls off "that hat trick" better than he does. She works as many hours and yet when she gets home she is able to get excited as the children tell her what happened to them during the day. Cary marvels at the way she musters the energy to interact with the children. "But then," he laments, "she's never interested in making love. I guess working and being with the kids is enough for her."

Marital tensions play a big part in Cary's mood. He and his wife may need to see a couple therapist. My hypothesis is that Cary is depressed because he is stuck in an untenable position and does not know what he can do to alter the situation. I ask him what he thinks might be stuck in his marriage. He guesses that he and Sarah might be engaged in a power struggle. I ask him what powers they each wield. He says he knows that she feels very inadequate on account of her inability to be sexually available and responsive, so he uses her sexual unavailability as an excuse for not listening to her when she wants to talk about how hard it is to have a career and a family. He guesses she uses the issue of shared domestic responsibilities to make him feel guilty:

"I never seem to be able to do enough. No matter how much housework I do, she stays up later finishing up. And yesterday she got angry at me and screamed that she doesn't even tell me all the times she has to wash the dishes or arrange childcare for the kids in order to cover for me when I forget to take care of things."

Reacting to what he considers a guilt trip, he turns a deaf ear when she wants to talk about her feelings. She uses guilt, he is passive–aggressive; an even match.

The Capacity to Confront a Partner and Work Through Relational Tensions

Tom avoids marriage like the plague. If asked, he would say it is because his mother was so intrusive and abusive that he does not want to find himself in another intimacy where there is no exit. This is not to say he is insensitive to women, nor unwilling to please. Quite the opposite, he is "the kind of man every woman would give her eye tooth for," or so he imagines. He is quite attractive to women. It is not only his looks and sparkling intelligence, he is also very sensitive and capable of talking about feelings. He is a therapist and employs his listening skills productively in his work. He was married in his mid-twenties and divorced after two years. And there have been two other primary relationships that have lasted as long. In one he and his lover lived together for one year, in the other he never lived with his partner. Besides these three relatively "long-term" relationships, Tom has dated hundreds of women. He is very proud of the fact that most women he dates say that he is the most emotionally available man they have ever met, that they admit sex is better with him than it has been with anyone else, and that they very soon want to make a commitment and eventually marry him.

"Then why have none of these relationships worked out?," I ask.

"I don't know. I always seem to get bored just when the woman begins to tell me she loves me. I get attracted to somebody else. I've just never been able to be monogamous, and none of the women I've been with could stand for that."

It frightens Tom that women keep telling him they feel a deep connection with him. He feels like he is deceiving them. He knows how to talk about feelings, and he is a good listener. But he admits he developed these skills as a teenager because he knew women were more likely to have sex with a sensitive man. He does not respect women who fall for him, but their willingness to be vulnerable and their praise for his sexual virtuosity make him feel powerful. He thinks he is "addicted" to admiration from women. He is seeking therapy because he is depressed. He has been thinking about having children but he does not believe he has ever been in love and wonders if he is capable of sustaining a committed relationship.

Psychoanalysts tell us that our adult romantic relationships are shaped by the kinds of relationships each partner once had with his or her parents, and that men and women regularly project their internalized images of parents onto their partners, causing the other to join him or her in acting out precisely the kinds of scenes that might have occurred in the childhood homes of one partner or the other (Meissner, 1978). I ask Tom why he has never considered the possibility that, by trying to resolve differences between himself and his partner, he might create a relationship that is more rewarding than the earlier one with his mother. Tom is able to admit he is afraid that if he marries he will be locking himself into a relationship with someone who, like his mother, might ignore his feelings and needs and bombard him with hers, just as his ex-wife did. And he is able to see that, by being so willing to listen to the women he dates while refusing to expose his vulnerabilities and needs, he repeatedly sets up a scenario wherein his partner seems to be overly needy and demanding, as if to fulfill his prophecy.

Why is it so hard for this man, and so many others, to trust that by actively processing conflicts with a woman, or a male partner, he will be able to attain a quality of intimacy he has not known in the past? There is a personal answer to that question, a different answer in every man's life; in Tom's case it is because he was never able to accomplish much improvement in a toxic relationship with his mother. There are also sociocultural factors. With sexual freedom, media portrayals of readily available sexy men and women (who seem forever young on account of working out at the right gym or drinking the right beer), the ease of "no-fault" divorce, the social stresses on marriages today (including the economic downturn that makes so many men subject to feelings of inadequacy), it should be no surprise that so many men and women choose to toss aside their marital vows instead of working very hard with a long-term partner to fix what ails the relationship.

There are male foibles that predispose to impasses in a primary intimacy (there are female foibles as well, but that is not the topic here). Consider, for instance, the man's unwillingness to admit the ways he depends on the woman, leaving her to wonder if she is the only one with dependency needs. Perhaps, if he could admit his dependency—for instance his need for constant reassurance from her that he is the one she loves and depends on—she might feel less the needy one. Then she might be able to come out of her depression and pay more attention to his emotional needs.

Sometimes the personal idiosyncrasies are so deep-seated and complicated that they are not very amenable to change. Some men refuse to permit much intimacy to develop with a woman because they are afraid of the rejection or betrayal they believe is inevitable. Other men avoid intimacy because they are afraid that when they get close to a woman the ugly side of their personality will emerge and they will abuse their partner or themselves and begin to drink heavily, for example. Women have idiosyncrasies too. Sometimes both partners are so wounded that it is hard for them to even begin the process of communication to work out their differences.

Sandy and Rochelle are unable to argue with each other without getting into a screaming match. They are in their late thirties and have been together for three years. She very much wants to have a child but he is ambivalent about it. He comes to see me seeking individual psychotherapy. He says he loves her very much but is unable to stand up to her. As a child, he was abused severely by alcoholic parents. His father beat his mother frequently, and both parents turned on him at the slightest provocation. There was always a pretense. Perhaps he spilled a glass of milk or slammed a door too hard. And the beatings began as "a spanking." His parents used a strap, but inevitably they moved on from spanking to whipping him on the shoulders and back as he crouched in a corner or tried to flee from the room.

Sandy remembers asking himself as a child what he had done to deserve this kind of punishment. And he always arrived at an answer: he was too noisy, too clumsy or "in the way." The last was a recurrent theme. He was an only child and his parents often talked about the freedom they might have had were it not for his unplanned birth. He remembers feeling that he was the sole cause of his parents' misery, and therefore the violence that erupted between them as well as the beatings he received really were his fault.

Children quite regularly accept this kind of blame. The reason is simple. If a very young child is treated badly, there are two ways for him or her to understand the situation. If the child concludes that the fault lies in the parents' badness, and the child has no way to change the parents, then the situation is quite bleak and the helpless child is at the mercy of those bad parents. If, on the other hand, the child concludes that there is something he or she is doing wrong and this is the cause of the abuse, then there is always the possibility that the child can change what he or she is doing and then the parents will change their behavior, take better care of the child, and the hellish situation will be abated. The child begins blaming himself or herself at a very young age and develops the habit of blaming him or herself in each ensuing situation. Even when, as an adult, the individual who has this kind of habit recalls childhood abuses, there is the lingering belief he or she really was at fault. Then, when blamed by a contemporary partner, whether the blame is warranted or not, the individual who has this habit will accept more than his or her share of the blame.

Rochelle's father deserted the family when she was quite young. She was the older of two sisters. She remembers angry battles with her mother, though there was no physical abuse. First her mother would be nice to her, for instance buying her a pretty dress, and then the older woman would turn against her and attack her for getting the dress dirty. The pattern continued as Rochelle began dating in her mid-teens. First her mother would encourage her to go out and meet boys, then when she managed to go on a date her mother would criticize her upon her return home, accusing her of being promiscuous or saying that it was insensitive for her to keep her mother awake worrying about her while she stayed out late.

Sandy and Rochelle had an intense and troubled relationship. They alternated between highs of passionate love and lows of bitter animosity. She would tell him that he was "the love of her life" and the only man who had ever truly understood her, and then she would proceed to insult and humiliate him in front of others. Once she acted quite seductive with a friend of his at a party. When he complained and began to leave the party by himself, she stopped him and insisted he take her home. During the drive home she teased him and said his jealousy was unmanly. On another occasion she told him he was not aggressive enough sexually, and then when he became more aggressive she stopped him and called him a brute and a rapist.

Both partners tend to alternate between two different states of mind. At one moment he is the admirable, caring man who deserves to be called the "love of her life," at another moment he is a despicable cad who deserves abuse and humiliation. At one moment she is the loving and lovable enchantress, and at another she is the angry, evil "slut." Both of the partners have trouble keeping in mind, when they are in one or the other split-off state of mind, that there is another side to them. He cannot keep in mind, when she is abusing him, that he is a lovable man who deserves respect and appreciation. At that moment, a captive of his childhood habit, he accepts her abuse and assumes he is a despicable character who deserves to be treated that way. At another moment he feels that things are grand, that he is deservedly the love of her life, and he barely remembers the bad moments.

Sandy needs to reclaim the aggression he buried as a child out of fear he would be killed by his parents if he fought back when they were attacking him. In addition, he swore from a very tender age never to be as abusive as his parents were, and since he has never been able to figure out how to stand up for himself without being a brute, this resolution has motivated him to bury his aggressive strivings even deeper. Unconsciously, he fell for Rochelle in part because he identified with her aggressiveness. In other words, while he could not permit himself to be aggressive he could vicariously enjoy his partner's forcefulness. She, meanwhile, acts out with him what her mother did to her. Thus, when he does begin to stand up to her she humiliates him, just as her mother humiliated her every time she began to make progress.

Sandy must reclaim the aggressive strivings he has been suppressing since childhood and learn to stand up to Rochelle and say with some conviction:

"Hey, wait a minute, I don't deserve to be treated that way, and if you don't begin to treat me better I'm not going to remain in this relationship very long."

She, on the other hand, must learn that he will not attack her as her mother did just when she makes herself most vulnerable, so she does not have to keep destroying the love that is growing between the two. In other words, if this couple is to learn to build a more consistently loving relationship, both must stand up to the other as whole individuals demanding to be treated decently.

Is It Different for Gay Couples?

While heterosexual couples enjoy the blessings of society, gay men, lesbians, and gay couples suffer the consequences of widespread homophobia and institutional discrimination. Gay couples are denied official marriage, shared health insurance, and joint tax returns. They are faced with huge legal obstacles when they try to adopt children, when the partner of the natural father seeks official recognition as a stepparent, when they seek paternity leave, and when it comes time to establish each partner's legitimate heirs. Society withholds approval and makes it very difficult for gay men to sustain committed primary relationships. Then there is the omnipresence of AIDS, the risk for both partners as well as the likelihood that the couple will lose many friends from the disease.

There are personal obstacles as well. Most gay men were raised by heterosexual couples and received little training in same-sex intimacies. Then, when both partners are men, there is a double dose of male foibles. So gay couples must be trailblazers. They must make room for compromise, otherwise how would they be able to avoid the kinds of battles that regularly erupt between men living in close quarters? And the partners cannot rely on a difference in gender to determine their respective roles and privileges. Who will take care of the house? Who will be the major provider? In sexual matters, Who is to be on top and who on the bottom? Who is to be active and who passive?

Straight couples may not follow tradition in every respect, but at least they have the tradition to bounce off of as they create their own path. Gay couples, from the beginning, must negotiate on a large number of issues that straight couples take for granted. As Laura Markowitz (1991) points out:

> The fact that same-sex couples have to balance stress in so many systems at once—their own families of origin, their relationship,

the gay/lesbian community, their ethnic or religious communities, and mainstream society—makes their efforts at forming a family an impressive juggling act. And the complexity of a relationship between people with the same gender socialization can create further confusion and conflict, yet the problem may not be evident to the straight therapist. (p. 33)

Then, in addition to the difficulties that confront gay couples in this society, there are also the kinds of tensions that creep into heterosexual relationships: the inevitable power struggles, jealousies, misunderstandings, and conflicts about autonomy vs. dependence. It is not easy to make a relationship work.

Adversity can intensify a couple's commitment and deepen the intimacy. Many long-term gay couples are realizing this and creating new forms of family life (Marcus, 1988). And we see evidence of the fruits of adversity in the way the gay community has responded to the AIDS epidemic with new ways to love and nurture terminally ill men.

Sex, Potency and Ambition

In David Lodge's (1975) *Trading Places*, Philip and Desiree have this conversation while lying naked in bed. He begins:

"You don't think it's on the small side?"
"It looks fine to me."
"I've been thinking lately it was rather small."
"A recent survey showed that ninety per cent of American men
    think their penises are less than average size."   .
"I suppose it's only natural to want to be in the top ten per cent.
    . . ." (p. 167)

While working with a man who complains of sexual dysfunction—impotence and premature ejaculation are the most frequent complaints—I assume that the sexual problem is a continuation in the bedroom of a more general and pervasive conflict, but the problem only seems obvious and upsetting when it surfaces and causes dysfunction in relation to sex. Of course, I only make this assumption once I have ruled out medical causes of sexual dysfunction, for instance chronic illnesses such as diabetes, vascular, and neurological conditions, and the side effects of antihypertensive and antidepressant medications.

Consider the problem of premature ejaculation. The first thing to note is the man's definition of premature. What standard is he employing to assess prematurity? Is the standard the time he imagines a potent man is capable of continuous intercourse? Is the standard his partner's satisfaction? Is he more intent on performing than he is on enjoying sexual encounters? Are inadequacy and shame part of the picture? How much performance anxiety is there? Does the man take full responsibility for the problem or does he see it as a relational difficulty?

Jed is a factory worker in his early thirties who has been married for three years to Martha. He enters psychotherapy complaining of premature ejaculation. As we explore his sexual difficulty it becomes clear there is more to the problem than the mechanics of ejaculation. He is aware that it takes a long time for his wife to reach orgasm, and complains that she is very demanding during their love-making, insisting he do a long list of things to her "because that's the only way I can come." In love-making, it seems, he caters to her needs and whims with very little reciprocity, and she complains that he has not done enough.

I ask if it would be fair to say their relationship is like that in other regards. He thinks about my question for awhile and responds in the affirmative.

"She does kinda call the shots most of the time. She has strong opinions, and if I insist on anything too much we get into a fight. Besides, it's not important to me anyway, and I'm glad to be able to make her happy."

In other words, sex is not the only arena in which Jed ignores his needs while taking care of Martha's. Of course, there is a power struggle as well. She is controlling. While he seems to be granting her total control, his refusal to wait for her to have an orgasm before he has one gives him another kind of control. And the symptom serves to express some of his anger and wish to frustrate her.

I point out to Jed that the sexual problem is not due to any deficiency in him, it is a relational issue. I suggest that, for a while, he and Martha reorganize their sexual encounters so that they are less serious about the goal of orgasm, there is more playfulness, intercourse is not the main activity, and they try to tell each other in words what they want the other to do to them. In addition I suggest that the timing of his orgasm become her responsibility. If she would like for him to wait longer, then she must notice when he is about to ejaculate and halt whatever they are doing. I suggest he set up this altered routine by first telling her that he really needs her help if he is to solve his sexual problem, and that he tell her she will probably need some practice figuring out when he is about to ejaculate.

Jed talks to Martha and they agree to try the plan. He reports a few weeks later that there is some improvement in his ability to delay ejaculation, but the main thing that has changed is that the couple is talking more about both partners' sexual desires, they are spending more time making love, and Martha says she actually prefers paying attention to his sexual needs—she had always felt uncomfortable about the fact he never let her know what he wanted her to do. Meanwhile, he has been taking more initiative in making other kinds of decisions and reports he feels less depressed.

When I ask Jed why he had never told Martha what he wanted her to do while they were making love, he responds that he believed she should just figure that out without his having to say anything.

"Do you feel that way about other things?" I ask.

"Well, yes, I guess I do. Martha comes home and starts talking about what's going on with her, and she just goes on and on. She never asks how my day has been."

"So why don't you just tell her?"

"If she were interested, she'd ask. And I don't want to be telling her about all that happened and spilling my guts and then find out she isn't even interested. That would just kill me!"

"Has that happened?"

"Yeah, a lot of times."

It turns out Jed's mother was very inattentive. She would ask him how his day had gone at school and then, before he had a chance to complete a sentence, she would leave the room and begin doing something else. I began to wonder if Martha was as inattentive and self-absorbed as Jed would have me believe, so I suggested he talk with her about this problem. He did, and returned the next week to inform me that she was surprised by his question, admitted that when he did not volunteer anything she tended to talk about herself, but claimed that she would be very interested in hearing from him about how his day had gone or what was on his mind. I pointed out the similarity between this exchange and the one about sexual cravings. In both cases he was surprised by the fact that, when he finally did state his needs, he found Martha very willing to hear them and respond.

Sexual impotence, when it is functional and not caused by an organic condition, is usually a symptom of a more pervasive male malaise. Since a man's sense of potency is rooted in his accomplishments and status, failure can lead to impotence. Sy, a married man in his early forties and the father of three young children, entered therapy because of severe depression, insomnia, and impotence of a few months' duration. He had been employed as a community organizer in a grass roots organization for fifteen years. Before that he and his wife of seventeen years had been active in the civil rights and antiwar movements.

Sy's oldest child had been attacked recently by a bully at the local public school. In discussing their child's dilemma, he and his wife arrived at the possibility that they might have to pull him out of the public school and enroll him in a private one. They quickly dismissed that idea because of the expense. But, in the weeks that followed, his wife continued to worry about the son's safety and the quality of his education, and this led to her depression, her self-castigation focusing on the couple's limited earning power. In reaction to his wife's depression, and her criticism of him for being unable to provide real financial security, this man fell into a deep depression and a troubling impotence.

The couple had a particularly painful argument one evening after putting the children to bed. She was alternatingly tearful and enraged as she exclaimed:

"If it weren't for your goddamn fear of success you'd have finished graduate school and gotten a decent job and I wouldn't have to work so hard—then I could spend more time with the kids and even do some of the writing I've always wanted to do!"

At first he argued that the community organizing he was doing was important. Then he broke down and cried too. He told me it was at that moment that he suddenly realized he'd been wasting his life. He had watched all the others he worked with in the community move on to graduate school and higher paying jobs. But by now it was too late for him. He was too old to go back to school, too old to be hired for an entry level job in a big company. By the time he entered therapy he was getting only one or two hours of sleep per night, spending the rest of the night thrashing about in bed obsessing about job opportunities he had turned down years before, and worrying about the family's financial straits. He had also become impotent. He saw no way out of his predicament, and said he would seriously consider suicide if it were not for the kids.

Interestingly, in the course of five or six weekly sessions where he obsessed about the impossibility of radically altering his situation at this late date and berated himself for all his inadequacies, he never once mentioned that there was another reason he had chosen to be a community organizer for a small organization that could not pay him a high salary or offer him much opportunity for advancement. That reason was his commitment to the aims of the community organiza-tion. The paid job had been a way to make a career of the kind of political work he had done as a young adult with no remuneration.

Conflicts about ambition play a central role in the male midlife crisis. For those who are satisfied with their accomplishments, midlife is a time to slow down and attend to undeveloped sides of the personality. But men who are dissatisfied tend to feel a failure, envy others, and sink into depression. When a man has always tried to put his ideals and his principles into practice in his everyday life and, on account of his principles, has missed opportunities for personal advancement, he might experience some regrets at midlife (Kupers, 1990).

In this case it was true that some of Sy's inner conflicts about performance and success had held him back. But that was only part of the picture. He had also firmly ascribed to certain principles. For instance, as a young adult he believed that he should not be paid a higher salary than others just because his family was affluent enough to send him to college. And part of his community organizing work involved helping disadvantaged youth go to college. In his depressive crisis Sy was focusing exclusively on his failings and his wife's unhappiness. He was ignoring the other side of the coin: his rather impressive success as a husband and father, the respect he had in the community as a commited organizer for important causes, and the integrity of a life created out of lived principles. Once he was able to shift his focus to include what was admirable about his life his depression lifted, he was able to make love with his wife, and the two of them were able to begin talking about what realistic moves they might make as a family to eventually allow her to do her writing and him to be more successful in his work.

Not all men's sexual difficulties are as amenable to therapeutic intervention as these two proved to be, and not all couples are as motivated to change. But these vignettes illustrate the way sexual problems can offer a window into the overall dynamics of relationships.

Beneath the Cloak of Gender Equality

Quite a few couples are attempting to live according to the principle of gender equality. This does not mean the two partners in a heterosexual couple have to be and do exactly the same things. In fact, the couples who are most successful at sustaining a mutually satisfying intimacy are the ones who can differentiate themselves while still maintaining the sense that neither is losing out on account of the arrangements. The notion of dividing every item of housework exactly in half is no longer the ideal, if it ever was a particularly useful aim. Most couples I know who once tried to share housecleaning, cooking, laundry, home repairs, car maintenance, and decisions about interior design have moved on to a give-and-take arrangement whereby each partner specializes in the things that he or she does best or prefers the most. Kitty Moore talks about partners being "captains of different ships" (1992, personal communication). For some couples gender reversals work, the father likes staying home with the young children while the mother prefers to work long hours in order to further her career. The question is not how absolutely perfect the split in relation to each area of responsiblity, but rather whether either partner feels oppressed by the way labors and benefits are divided.

It is not easy for a couple to establish equitable gender roles. There is the social reality that men, on the average, have more earning capacity than women. There is "the feminization of poverty," the fact that there are more poor, single women who head households than there were prior to the Women's Movement (Pearce, 1978). Then there is "the second shift," the reality that in the average intact marriage where both partners work the woman tends to do more of the housework (Hochschild, 1989). Diane Ehrensaft (1987) points out that even in families in which the parents agree to strive toward equal co-parenting, women tend to initiate more than their share of the childrearing responsibilities and end up being the one who checks that things are done. Anne Bernstein (1989) studies stepfamilies and discovers that even if the mother is the stepparent she ends up initiating more than her share of parental interventions, while men, when they are the stepparent, feel more justified in stepping back and letting the natural mother do more. In other words, unnoticed or unspoken gender inequities continue, even in conscientious couples striving to attain equality. On the average, the man is more likely not to notice, the woman more likely not to mention it.

An additional problem is that a man might consciously ascribe to certain principles while his unconscious conflicts lead him to violate those principles. I mentioned the marriage of Cary and Sarah. Several months after the beginning of individual psychotherapy, Cary appeared for a session quite distraught and announced that he hit Sarah over the weekend. They argued, she pushed him, and he hit her with a closed fist on the back of her head. He was shocked that he had done it, and so was she. He tells me he wants to quit therapy because we are not getting at the deeper issues, the ones that led to his violence. He is ashamed of what he did, and was thinking of not coming to see me because it would be too embarassing to talk about it.

Cary and I agree the situation is serious, and he says he will stop procrastinating and go with his wife to see a couple therapist. Meanwhile, there are some issues he and I can discuss. Having agreed that it is not O.K. for him to hit his wife no matter how much she provokes him, he resolves not to do it again and we begin to explore the sources of his anger. The thing that bothered him the most was her refusal to acknowledge how much time he had been spending with the kids while she was working night and day on a project at her office. She yelled that she shouldn't have to acknowledge his pitching in with the kids since he never acknowledges all the extra things she regularly does for the kids and for him. The shoving began and he hit her.

Cary feels he gives away too much power:

"It's been that way from the beginning. She wanted to get married so I went along. She wanted to have kids. I would have eventually initiated it, but she was ready to have kids long before I would have been, and I went along. And I have always been willing to cut back my hours at work to take on more things at home so she could work. Now I'm glad we've done all these things, don't get me wrong, but there have been sacrifices. All I want is a little acknowledgment. Is that too much to ask?"

I ask Cary what he gets for being so good. He tells me it just makes him feel good. When Sarah smiles and tells him how great it is of him to do so much at home, he feels like he "walks very tall." I ask him if there is any reason for him to be needing more of that kind of feedback from her right now. He thinks it might be because he is feeling inadequate at work, an important project is turning out to be a failure, he is losing a client, and his confidence is suffering. I question him about his definition of manliness and he begins to describe a man who overcomes immense obstacles in order to accomplish something great. We compare his assessment of himself and discover that he does not qualify.

"I know, if I would only value the things I do well—dividing my energies between work and home, raising kids who have their heads on straight, and supporting my wife to be all she can be—then I'd think of myself as a successful man. But it's hard to think like that when I'm all alone with my thoughts and I'm realizing how mediocre my work is."

As Cary recites his list of manly virtues, notice he disqualifies the man who puts ambition on the back burner while he stays home with the kids and supports his wife's career aspirations. He thinks about his father, who gave up a high-level managerial job because it would have required that the family move to another city. Then his father was laid off from the company he had worked for for eighteen years and went into a severe depression. His mother took charge at home and told the kids to go easy on their father. He remembers how angry he was at his father for needing "to hide behind a woman's skirt." Somehow the topic shifts to Cary's recent fight with Sarah, and he is able to examine his rage from a different perspective.

Cary was afraid that by giving up some of his own career aspirations he was becoming less of a man. Sarah's failure to acknowledge his sacrificies made him doubly angry. In addition, he felt that in the act of shoving him she was mocking his commitment to principle. For instance, she thought he would not hit her back because of the principle a man is never supposed to hit a woman no matter what the provocation. She was taking advantage of his commitment to that principle when she shoved him, and he felt mocked for his principled stance.

"Suddenly I felt like I was my father, the one everyone mocked in our family. So I lost it and let her have it!"

Cary and Sarah went to see a couple therapist. He vowed never to hit her again and they were able to discuss the importance of *mutual* acknowledgment in their relationship.

The Shoulds That Constrict, The Shame That Isolates

Whether it is the wish for a larger penis or the mandate to be at the top of the hierarchy, men feel burdened by the "shoulds" that they learned while undergoing training for manhood. Men "should" stand tall, take care of others without displaying too much softness, keep emotions contained, and avoid tears where possible. When a man is unable to carry out all the shoulds, he feels inadequate, there is shame, and then he isolates himself, making it more difficult to resolve the tensions in interpersonal relationships.

A young unmarried couple who had been living together for several years went on a vacation and rented a cabin by a lake. A man followed the woman as she was returning from the lake, forced his way into the cabin, pulled a gun, tied the male partner up, and proceeded to rape the woman. The intruder escaped. The couple, quite traumatized, returned home. In the weeks that followed he insisted that she not tell people about what had happened because it was too humiliating for him. The woman eventually went to see a therapist complaining of depression. It quickly became clear that the isolation her partner was imposing on her in order to avoid his shame was preventing her from getting the support she needed from others to work through the trauma she had undergone. She resolved to confront her partner and insist on her right to tell their friends about the rape. Her partner was then forced to confront his shame and look at the way he was isolating himself instead of seeking the support he needed. He eventually figured out that some of the "shoulds" he was laboring under were totally unrealistic. And she figured out that by putting aside her needs in order to protect him she was condemning herself to irresolution and depression. In fact, when the couple told their friends what had happened there was an immediate outpouring of sympathy and support, and both partners began to feel better.

Notice the male theme as it surfaces in this story. The man on top is strong, virile, and able to protect his female partner. If he fails to protect a partner, he is not only a weakling and a loser, but also feels shame on account of his failure and consequently feels he must isolate himself rather than sharing his pain with others. Shame and isolation form a vicious cycle; the more shame a man feels, the stronger the urge to be isolated. This vicious cycle is quite counterproductive in the context of a primary intimacy, especially when the partner wants to know what the man is feeling and to help him cope with his pain.

Lillian Rubin (1983) interviewed 150 couples from around the country and found that most couples are confused by recent changes in gender roles and gender relations. According to Rubin, some changes are easier than others: "The redistribution of household chores and other domestic arrangements, for example, requires only that there are two people of good will, good intention, and a willingness to engage the issue." Other issues go deeper and are more difficult to change, for instance, "how we handle our dependency needs, or how we express our needs for both intimacy and distance" (p. 206).

Gordon and Meth (1990) comment:

> Men today are caught between the old and the new, between holding onto the breadwinner role and trying to share more. The "old" values husbands learned from their fathers and the "new" ones introduced by their wives and the socioeconomic changes in family life are frequently not in concert. (p. 67)

Men are caught between the lessons they learned from their fathers—including the unverbalized one that raising children is woman's work—and the current reality of mothers who work and fathers who co-parent. How is a man to know what is the manly thing to do? No wonder so many men attend men's events designed to explore what it means to be a man.

Rubin shares a personal anecdote. She and her husband very consciously decided to create a role-reversal. He had been supporting her while she went to graduate school, but he wanted to quit his job and devote all his time to writing, a switch that would greatly decrease his income. After she graduated they agreed that he would quit his job and she would assume the major responsibility for supporting the family while he devoted more time to writing. She reports that a month or two after the switch he fell into a deep depression and she found herself getting furious at him. Rubin writes:

> He struggled with his sense of failure, with the fear that somehow his very manhood had been damaged. I—the liberated, professional woman—was outraged and enraged that he wasn't taking care of me any longer. I felt as if he had violated some basic contract with which we had lived, as if he had failed in his most fundamental task in life—to keep me safe and cared for, to protect and support me. (p. 23)

In other words, the man's depression and the woman's fury were signs that some very old "shoulds" were still in effect.

In my own case, the shoulds took over during a construction project. My wife and I, in partnership with two women friends, purchased some land in the country several years ago. We decided to build a cabin on the land and decided we would be partial owner-builders. We purchased plans and some prefabricated sections of the cabin; then we hired carpenters, plumbers, and electricians and planned to work alongside them. In addition, we asked some friends to come and help with the building.

One of our women partners took the lead and began to enquire of the men who lived in the vicinity how to accomplish the various tasks that were required if we were to get moving on the construction. Our male neighbors were eager to assist the women builders. They must have thought my partners' complete lack of expertise was cute, and must have enjoyed the opportunity to help. But where did that leave me? I found myself in the position of needing to ask these neighbors how to do things—from buying materials to replacing frozen pipes—that I secretly felt I should already know how to do. All along I wondered if the men would think I was a total wimp, but on each occasion, when I took a deep breath and proceeded to ask for help, they turned out to be friendly and nonjudgmental.

Then the time arrived for intensive on-site construction. Half of the friends we invited were men, one was a carpenter-contractor, and one of the women was a carpenter. As we began to build I found myself, the single male owner-builder, among people who knew much more than I did about every aspect of the project. Inwardly I felt some shame. As a man I "should" take charge and know what to do (my women partners, including my wife, were not saddled with this particular should). But as we moved from task to task—framing, sheetrocking, the installation of plumbing fixtures and so forth—I repeatedly found I did not know what to do and someone else took over. Between the partners' families there were seven teenage boys involved in the building process, and they were quite willing to take instruction from anyone who knew what to do. Again, I felt I "should" be able to instruct them, but repeatedly I had to tell them to ask someone else how to proceed. It turned out that I worked most on the roof, by myself, as if in nailing roofing tiles I was constructing a safety barrier between myself and the people and problems that remained down below.

After we finished building the cabin and returned home, Arlene and I had a vicious argument, punctuated by screaming matches that went on for several days. Eventually we spent several hours talking to another couple about our fight and were able to find grounds for a tentative resolution of our differences. (We feel very fortunate to have a couple we trust and with whom we can trade unofficial "therapy sessions" whenever serious tensions develop in either marriage.) One of the things we figured out was that I had felt ashamed of not being able to lead the construction team. I felt I was failing to be the "hero" whom the "damsel" could depend on in her moment of distress, so I withdrew from her in shame. She did feel some anger toward me for not taking charge, and she agreed that piece of the puzzle might involve her conflicts about rapidly changing gender roles and relations, but she was even angrier that I had failed to stay in better contact with her so we could help each other through what had been a strange and difficult experience for both of us. Instead of working together, we had become alienated. I accepted much of the blame for that; isolation was my way of coping with the shame I felt when I could not fulfill an unrealistic set of "shoulds."

Forward Motion

When Martha first agreed to take responsibility for the timing of Jed's orgasms, she was merely complying with his wishes. But soon she realized there were benefits for her in the plan to have her pay more attention to his sexual and emotional needs, for instance, there would be less cause for guilt about her being self-indulgent and controlling. Similarly, the man whose partner was raped was at first merely bowing to her wishes when he agreed to talk to their friends about the traumatic incident. But when he discovered that talking, far from aggravating his shame, helped him cope with his feelings, he admitted he had learned something valuable as a result of his partner's demand. And I was eventually able to see that Arlene's complaint about my isolating myself during the construction project was not only valid, it was also a valuable lesson on how to cope with my shame in stressful situations.

There is a two-step process that occurs in couples who are willing to learn from each other during and after the upheavals that punctuate their relationship. First one partner bows to the other's demand; second the resulting change in the way the partners relate turns out to be an improvement, even in the eyes of the partner who originally only complied in order to keep the peace. If the second step does not follow the first, the partner who gave in is likely to resent how much he or she repeatedly has to back down in order to make the relationship work, and the unspoken resentment that lingers after the resolution of one squabble will already contain the seeds of the next major squabble. Of course, there must be open discussion between the partners if there is to be forward motion in the relationship, and it is especially helpful if the partners are able to openly acknowledge how much they have learned from each other.

CHAPTER 5

Pornography and Intimacy

Feminists are engaged in a rancorous debate. According to the antipornography side, pornography fosters violence against women by publicly displaying images of women being objectified and violated. Robin Morgan (1980) claims: "Pornography is the theory, and rape is the practice." Andrea Dworkin (1989) believes that men have committed atrocities throughout history because of their "sexual obsession":

> Pornography reveals that slavery, bondage, murder, and maiming have been acts suffused with pleasure for those who committed them or who vicariously experienced the power expressed in them. (p. 69)

Susan Griffin (1981) describes pornography as "the mythology of the male chauvinist mind" (p. 2).

The other side does not refute the fact that the pornography industry, as a whole, promotes sexism—it would be rather difficult to do so and still call oneself a feminist—but argues that a dogmatic stance against all forms of pornography merely sets up an alternative form of censorship and social control. In other words, where patriarchs have for centuries set themselves up to prescribe and proscribe acceptable forms of sexuality for women, some feminists would substitute their improved, nonsexist prescriptions and proscriptions for everyone. How is one to evaluate the implications—for gender politics—of two lesbians privately enjoying a video of two women engaged in sadomasochistic acts?

The debate touches on civil liberties. In taking a stand against pornography, are feminists aligning themselves with rightwingers who would censor all graphic sexual portrayals? What of Robert Maple-thorpe's work? His photos are considered erotic by some and pornographic by others. The latter would preclude galleries from showing his work and, using Maplethorpe as an example, would cut off public grants to artists they consider pornographic. According to Kate Ellis (1990):

> Anti-porn feminism has made our proposed revolution unappeal-ing even to some of us who want such a revolution. (p. 434)

Gayle Rubin (1981) writes:

> Of course, I'm against violence against women. But I don't feel that I can express my politics towards the violence against women, because the only form in which a politics opposed to violence against women is being expressed is anti-sexual. (p. 51)

Ilene Philipson (1990) regrets that the debate ends up pitting the "good girls" who would suppress pornography against the "bad girls" who would fight to prevent any encroachment on their sexual freedom. And Lorna Weir and Leo Casey (1990) convincingly argue that the whole debate is ill-conceived: "We reject both these positions... from a perspective that values a plurality of ethical sexualities, excluding only those practices that have been established through democratic discussion as coercive or violent" (p. 461).

The debate raises questions for progressive men. Some are eager to join the antipornography bandwagon by clearly distinguishing their own intentions from those of sadists, rapists, pornographers, and other misogynists. John Stoltenberg (1989) argues that pornography institu-tionalizes and eroticizes male supremacy:

> We've got to be telling other men that if you let the pornographers lead you by the nose (or any other body part) into believing that women exist to be tied up and hung up and beaten and raped, it's not okay. (p. 135)

David Mura (1987) believes that the pornographer is really abusing himself, making himself one-dimensional and "stupid":

> A man wishes to believe there is a beautiful body with no soul attached. Because of this wish he takes the surface for truth. There are no depths. Because of this wish, he begins to worship an image. But when this image enters the future, it loses what the man has given it—momentary devotion. The man wishes for another body,

another face, another moment. He discards the image like a painting. It is no longer to his taste. Only the surface can be known and loved, and this is why the image is so easily exhausted, why there must be another (p. 66)

Men Against Pornography (1990), a group formed to struggle for sexual justice, has created a checklist for signs of addiction to pornography:

You become dissatisfied with your sexual partner's physical appearance or how they express themselves sexually; you need to remember images or scenes from pornography in order to have sex with someone; you withdraw into yourself or you become less outgoing; and so forth. (p. 294)

Taking the other side, Alex Rode Redmountain (1990) argues that he is a feminist, yet:

Like many of my friends, I still enjoy it. It turns me on and reminds me that I'm a sexual creature. It satisfies my curiosity about all the women I'll never be with. It has, I believe, made me a better lover, and it has certainly helped make me a more tolerant human being. (p. 77)

Bernie Zilbergeld (1990) claims pornography can be therapeutic to the extent it spices up sex lives and enhances marriages. Alan Soble (1986) wonders if the objectification of women is a necessary part of pornography, and whether in the future it might be possible to create nonsexist pornography—if there were to be truly democratic decisions about its content and uses.

Michael Kimmel (1990) has put together a rich anthology of men's attitudes about pornography—pro and con. In reviewing the literature, it seems to me that those who would justify the consumption of pornography tend to lose the forest for the trees; for instance, making absurd comments about disconnected fragments of the pornographic experience and missing the larger point of feminist protest. Thus, Phillip Lopate writes (1990): "The woman on the film screen is certainly undisturbed by the jets of sperm her beauty has inspired" (p. 29). Meanwhile, the clearest case against pornography comes from those who situate its consumption in a social context; for instance, Harry Brod (1988) argues:

Its commodification of the body and interpersonal relationships paves the way for the ever more penetrating ingression of capitalist market relations into the deepest reaches of the individual's psychological makeup. (p. 277)

I should be clear about where I stand in the ongoing debate. I will limit this discussion to pornography consumption among heterosexual men because there are different issues involved for women and gays. I believe the whole debate is based on overly broad generalizations. Where is the line to be drawn between pornography and art? Is it possible to explicitly depict heterosexual sex without objectifying women? Does it make a difference if a video is directed and produced by women or that a heterosexual couple selects a video that neither finds objectionable and consents to view it together? These details are rarely addressed by the debaters, as if there were no grey areas. Still, I believe the overall effect of pornography as a commercial industry is to foster the objectification of women, and hence the consumer of pornography is acting in complicity with a sexist industry even if it were possible to find a particular form of pornographic material and a viewing situation that are not entirely objectionable; but I do not believe the campaign to outlaw pornography will solve anything. Rather, I believe a campaign of public discussion and education, as well as political organization, is needed to combat the objectification of women by the pornography industry as well as by the media in general.

I see quite a number of men in psychotherapy who tell me they consume pornography. They also believe that the consumption of pornography is morally wrong, even oppressive toward women, and yet they still consume it. None of these men are wife-beaters, rapists or child-molesters. Why do they consume pornography? How do they justify it? These men are embarassed to admit that they resort to pornography, so it serves no useful purpose for me to lecture them on the morality and politics of their private acts; in fact, that would only make them feel worse. As a therapist, I listen without judging, and try to understand the problems in a man's life—they are almost always in the area of intimacy—that he believes will be solved by his resorting to pornography. What does their process in the consulting room teach us about ways to transcend the pornographic imagination?

Men Talk About Pornography in the Consulting Room

Gene seeks therapy because of depression. He tells me he supports his wife in her bid to do well in her profession, and he says they love each other and he would never do anything that might jeopardize the stability of their marriage. But she is not very interested in sex. For him, it is a big problem. It's not so much the sexual frustration—he satisfies himself while looking through porn magazines—it's that he needs to feel more passion in his marriage.

Gene also complains that he feels depressed at work. His job is boring, but usually he finds solace in socializing with co-workers. Now he's feeling left out when his colleagues gather. He says he has "an odd notion" that they do not really like him. For instance, today at lunch he walked toward a table where four co-workers were sitting. He thought of pulling up a chair and squeezing in but decided that since they were talking so animatedly, they probably did not want anyone to intrude on the group. I ask what his problem in the lunchroom has to do with his wife and he explains that, when he feels good about his marriage—that is, when his wife is interested in sex and he feels desired—he feels more confident at work and will readily barge into a group engrossed in conversation, sometimes even taking over the group.

We discuss his dependence on his wife's attitude, the dangers of staking so much on her whims, and some ways he might prevent the feeling that he is unloved at home from spreading to relationships at work. Of course, his relationship with his mother figures prominently, and we examine the parallels. The topic shifts to his interest in pornography. Gene explains that he knows, on a conscious level, that his wife is not having an affair, but sometimes, in a "paranoid moment," he feels very much the cuckold. When he feels unlovable and paranoid he turns to pornography and masturbates.

"It helps me stop obsessing about the fact she's not turned on to me."

We also explore the possibility that his consumption of pornography might have something to do with the way he isolates himself at work while feeling it is the others who are actively excluding him.

"It does seem like that happens more right after I've been binging on porno magazines and masturbating a lot."

* * *

Richard is single. He was beaten as a child by an alcoholic father. He is quick to anger, and occasionally gets into fights in bars. He is afraid that he will be violent in a primary relationship, so he avoids women. He seeks psychotherapy asking if I can help him control his angry outbursts. We quickly uncover a pattern: he tends to fall for a woman very quickly, she is not as interested as he in establishing a committed relationship, he becomes violent and causes exactly what he wanted to avoid: she leaves him. In a couple of relationships he has actually hit his partner, "only slaps across the cheek," he quickly adds. He has resolved to live alone and resort to pornography whenever he gets horny. He explains to me that it's safer that way—no one gets hurt. Meanwhile, he is depressed. Not being able to really trust men, and not being able to stay with a woman, he feels very lonely.

*   *   *

Don, young for thirty, tells me that he and his lover of three years live separately because he has to have a lot of time to himself. I ask what he does when he is alone, and among his list of private activities is pornography. It turns out there is a pattern. He and his lover get very close during a three day weekend together, he begins to feel bored and decides they need to be apart for three or four days, he tells her he feels "too crowded" and then, once alone, and even if he is not feeling particularly sexual, he rents pornographic videos and masturbates. It is as if he were substituting pornographic women and onanism for his lover and their lovemaking. Pornography serves to create distance. Memories of the couple's weekend lovemaking fade into the background as he imagines sex with each of the women on the screen.

*   *   *

Mike knows he uses pornography to distance his wife. In fact, he is very clear about the pattern. He makes sexual advances, his wife rebukes him, and he figures she will be more interested the next night (if it's been awhile since they have made love, he feels "it's time"). Again she disappoints him. After a few disappointments he says to himself:

"Okay, I'll show her, when she starts craving sex I won't be available. I'll get a porno film and masturbate, then when she starts making advances I'll be unresponsive."

*   *   *

Jack is a timid man in his mid-twenties. He had never been in a long-term primary relationship until he met Sally a couple of years ago. He seeks therapy because he is quite worried that Sally will leave him, and yet he does not find their relationship very satisfying. We explore his concerns only to discover that for six months she has seemed uninterested in being with him, preferring to spend time at her workplace and with friends. He feels rejected.

Jack tells me during the second therapy session that he never really stands up to Sally, he is too afraid she will get upset and leave. A few sessions later he informs me that since adolescence he has enjoyed renting X-rated videos and masturbating. Though sex has always been "good" with Sally, he has continued to rent videos during the course of their relationship. I ask him if there is any identifiable time sequence in his use of videos. After pausing to think about the question he realizes that he usually rents a video when the couple is in the middle of a big argument.

When the couple fights, he feels he has to get away from her in order to avoid losing control of his anger and saying something he will regret—or hitting her. At such times he finds release in viewing a pornographic video and masturbating. After doing that for a few days, he usually finds that he is calm enough to return to Sally and attempt to resolve their differences.

What Attracts These Men to the Pornographic Woman?

The pornographic woman has advantages. Always available for a sexual encounter, she screams and moans with abandon. She is not shy about exposing her body to the man's gaze (Gene is unhappy about the fact that his wife refuses to undress in front of him and prefers to wear a tee shirt while making love). She never menstruates, nor is she concerned about sexually transmitted diseases. She makes no demands for a committed relationship, she is never sick nor uninterested in sex, her body is never marred by cancer surgery. She does not wrinkle or age in any discernable way, there is no menopause, and she is always very interested in pleasing a man. In other words, she is the perfect sex object.

She is familiar for another reason. She is an effective mirror for a man who wishes to see himself larger than life. She gets turned on instantly. The video viewer, after erasing from his mind the image on the screen of that other male figure with an erect penis, can imagine that he has aroused her to this height of passion. The pornographic woman can be, for a moment, the mirror that possesses "the magic and delicious power of reflecting the figure of man at twice its natural size" (Virginia Woolf, 1929). The man can retreat to a secret place where he uses a woman to enlarge his ego, and he does not have to cope with the real women in his life who would be offended by the one-sidedness of the mirroring.

Of course a sensitive man would never demand that his mate override her own moods and inclinations in order to be sexually available whenever he feels the urge. His sensitivity toward women prevents him from faulting her—consciously. But unconsciously he may be fuming. Some men have affairs with younger women, visit prostitutes (actually, much of what is said here about pornography and intimacy applies as well to men who resort to paying for sex instead of struggling with their partners to create a fulfilling sex life and primary intimacy) or switch partners frequently in order to avoid struggling with a woman around difficult issues. The men I have described would like to avoid infidelity and do not want to be Don Juan. But they are blocked in their attempts to struggle with their partners and use pornography as an escape. At least the pornographic woman, by writhing and moaning, can let a man know how much he is desired.

A Secret Place

It is frightening how easily men are able to split their time between the social place where a sensitive man tries not to devalue women and the secret place—in one's head as well as in the video booth—where the objectification of women is permissible. Men tend to split. (Pornography is not the only instance, it is simply illustrative.) The misogynist mentally undresses all women he encounters, harrasses all those over whom he has power, engages in destructive affairs, lies to lovers about his wife and lies to his wife about his secret life, and has the kind of marriage where neither partner bothers to search for the truth about the other any longer. More sensitive men are not as prone to harrass women and lie about affairs, so they try to find less objectionable ways to create distance in a relationship, and sometimes resort to pornography in that context. But the fact that a man goes to that secret place, and essentially leaves a part of himself there when he returns to his lover, means their intimacy cannot be complete. For instance, every time his partner asks him what is on his mind while he happens to be thinking about a pornographic image, he feels he must lie to her. The little lies accumulate until his partner begins to complain he is not really present in the relationship. And he is not.

Freud (1913b) enjoyed telling the story of the "free house," the point in a town where no arrests would be made, no matter what the crimes of people assembled there. "How long would it be before all the riff-raff of the town had collected there?" (p. 136). Pornography is like the free house: that secret place becomes the place where all secret thoughts go, and as the secrets accumulate there the quality of a primary relationship deteriorates. The man finds himself in an untenable position. On the one hand he would like to be open and tell his partner how he feels; on the other hand he is not at all certain she will be able to cope with his true feelings, for instance his dissatisfactions with their sex life. This is not to say there should be no secrets in a primary relationship, but when splitting and secret-keeping become compulsive and habitual, there is a limit to the quality of intimacy a couple can attain.

Men tend to tell their therapists what they cannot tell their mates, so I hear about wives who are overweight, "too tired all the time," menopausal, sick, or unattractive—but the husbands do not know how to discuss such things with their partners without seeming insensitive. Recently a man told me his wife is always suffering from one or another illness and is consequently uninterested in sex. He feels he cannot tell her how frustrated he is with her—because he believes that feedback would decimate her—so he turns to pornography. He believes pornography objectifies women and should be boycotted, but, on the other hand he thinks it may be the lesser of two evils in his situation. He tells me:

"If I didn't resort to pornography I would either get really angry at her for being so tired all the time or I would have an affair."

It is when men find themselves in an untenable situation that they are most likely to split. A situation is untenable when the man feels trapped, when every option he can imagine seems precluded for some reason and all he wants to do is escape. One man does not want to tell his wife that her obesity is turning him off sexually for fear she will never recover from the insult. Another man does not know what to do with the rage he feels toward his partner, since he believes a man should not vent his anger on a woman who is smaller than him and more likely to be hurt. A third man tells me that his wife demands he tell her what he is feeling, but when he tells her he is angry at her she responds by feeling guilty and getting depressed. He does not want to make his wife depressed, so he keeps his feelings to himself, but then there is little for the two of them to talk about so he avoids personal conversations altogether. Then she gets upset because he does not tell her what is on his mind. One avenue of escape is pornography. At least, while engaged in an imaginary sex act with a pornographic woman, a man does not have to worry about a troubled personal life. Joel Kovel (1990) describes pornography as "the erotic less its negativity, less its ambivalence, its association of sexuality with death, and, finally, its truthfulness" (p. 165).

The man who has a secret place in his mind where he is "stupid" (Mura, 1987) begins to suffer from a certain lack of vitality. Gene is depressed and Jack's relationship with Sally lacks passion. The dynamic that leads these men to the sex shop is circular: They complain about a lack of passion and sexual energy in their primary relationships, they turn to pornography in order to express their sexual and aggressive energies more on their own terms, and then they discover they cannot bring the energy generated by the pornographic experience back into their real relationship because they are hiding it in that secret place where they have imaginary sex with pornographic women.

The Psychotherapist's Stance vis à vis Pornography

Victor Seidler (1989) believes pornography is a roadblock on the path to deeper intimacy: "Because it is often the intimacy that we fear, many men turn to pornography, since this seems to offer the excitement without the personal vulnerability" (p. 163). To the extent a man uses pornography to flee from difficult tensions in a primary relationship, his consumption of pornography is a symptom. The therapist's task is to help him face what it is that makes him distance his partner. If the therapist is successful in helping the man resolve some of the conflicts that make his primary relationship unsatisfactory, then, in this specific case, the need to consume pornography should diminish.

At the start of the therapy, I do not take a stand for or against pornography. These men are exposing to me a sexual secret, which makes them vulnerable to feelings of shame. Why should I judge? I am not claiming that the therapist is neutral, just that, to begin with, something other than a lecture on morality is called for. If the therapist can listen carefully and help the client make some sense of the troubled intimacy, then work can begin on the inner conflicts that drive him to consume pornography.

Gene, Richard, Don, and Jack are all incapable of articulating their feelings and needs. Gene is unable to tell his wife he desires more passion in their marriage because he does not want to seem unsupportive of her efforts to build her career. Richard is so afraid of losing control and becoming violent with a woman that he cannot be sufficiently open about his feelings to make a relationship work. Don is unable to say to his partner that he needs to be alone at certain times, so he must live separately and resort to pornography in order to create distance. And Jack is unable to argue with Sally, turning instead to pornography to dilute their altercations.

Of course, part of the reason men have difficulty finding a tenable stance in their personal lives is that they feel they are being asked to be a new kind of man, one who is open about his feelings and very committed to family life, while still being expected to satisfy the traditional expectations, for instance, the expectation that a man be a good provider. Meanwhile, with the economic downturn, it is much more difficult to be a good provider. As one man explained to me after reporting that his wife was furious with him over the weekend because he does not make enough money to take the family on a vacation she had her heart set on:

"She can't have it both ways, I take time off from work to spend quality time with the kids, and then she rants and raves about my making less money; doesn't she understand that the guys who can afford to take their families on fancy vacations work ten hours a day, six days a week, and hardly ever see their kids except on vacations?"

All of these men are confused by the contradiction between their conscious espoused principles and their occasional lapses into fantasies and activities that are inconsistent with those principles. Pornography is not the only issue that that sets up this contradiction. Men are also alarmed to discover that they resent their childrearing and housekeeping responsibilities, or that they envy women their vitality and friendships. Many men actually are angry at the women in their lives whom they view as too independent and too powerful—angry because, on account of their independence, these women are not as available to satisfy a man's needs. But, rather than exploring difficult, painful issues with their partners, they escape into pornography.

Gene explains how he begins to find himself in an untenable situation:

"Then, when she is home and not involved with work or any of her friends and I make sexual advances, she begs off claiming she is not feeling well. She has allergies and is often not feeling well. How can I confront her and demand she be more turned on to me when she's sick? I'd have to be a real cad!"

So he turns to pornography instead. Gene and I agree it would be a good idea for him to find a way to talk with his wife about the issues that make him feel trapped in an untenable situation.

Don believes his lover is very sensitive about abandonment, and would be hurt if he were with her but not interested in relating. This is why he insists on living separately. I ask him to consider the possibility of discussing this whole dynamic with her (he does not have to confess to consuming pornography—that discussion may or may not eventually occur) to find a better way to work through the boundary between them. Perhaps, if he approaches the subject more effectively and she is able to see her part in making him feel engulfed, they can work out a better system for regulating their boundaries.

Susan Griffin (1981) offers a psychoanalytic interpretation of the pornographic scene wherein the woman is driven to madness by a desire to put a man's penis in her mouth, and the man holds back and frustrates her:

> This image reminds the mind of another scene, a scene in which this avidity to put a part of the body into the mouth is not a mystery. Here is a reversal again. For it is the infant who so overwhelmingly needs the mother's breast in his mouth. The infant who thought he might die without this, who became frantic and maddened with desire, and it was his mother who had the power to withhold. Now this reversal becomes, in and of itself, a humiliation. The mother is punished. She herself is made into an infant, and the hero can cooly grant or deny her frantic infant desire. (p. 61)

In other words, the boy grown into the pornographer gets back at the frustrating mother transformed into the pornographic woman—all unconsciously, of course. This is merely one of many possible psychodynamics.

The more rigidly men guard against all feelings and impulses that contradict their stated principles, the more force those urges gather as they sit in the unconscious waiting to burst through the barrier of repression. Warded off inclinations that violate consciously espoused principles are most likely to surface during moments of peak emotion, for instance, in the middle of a heated argument when a man finds it difficult to control the urge to hit his partner. The eruption frightens the man and he backs off. Then, in order to avoid losing control, he suppresses his rage and turns to pornography. Again, there is a vicious circle. The more he remains silent about his dissatisfactions and suppresses his anger, the more resentful he becomes. The point is reached where the resentment can no longer be contained; at least the man fears it cannot be contained, and this fear perpetuates the pattern.

Don complains his wife is intrusive. She seems to be very anxious to tap into his state of mind. As soon as he walks into the house after work, she greets him enthusiastically and asks how his day has been. At that moment, he just wants to sink into the sofa and relate to no one, but he does not explicitly tell her that. In response to her persistent questions, he produces grunts and curtailed comments. Eventually she backs off. Later, she wants to know whether or not he saw his therapist (me) today. He bluntly says it is none of her business. She is hurt; he does not respond. This continues until she can stand it no longer and wants to know if he is angry at her about something. He yells that he certainly is, it's her goddamn prying all the time. She gets up and runs to her room crying. Eventually he goes in to comfort her, and a peaceful calm results, neither talking much as they go on about their household routines.

We discuss the pattern. I ask if he and his wife are able to talk about their interactions. He admits that he does not want to talk to her about it because, for him, the act of talking would constitute his giving in—after all, it is she who desires more emotional contact, and if he gives her that while not getting what he wants from the exchange, he will feel humiliated. I am confused, and wonder out loud if Don is really this involved in a power struggle with his wife. He admits it is not really the issue of power that stops him at this point. He complains that, though his wife asks him to talk about his feelings, she is not really interested in hearing how he feels. She usually changes the subject just when he begins to talk about his feelings. He is afraid he will start talking about his feelings, she wil become disinterested and change the subject, and he will feel humiliated for having bothered to tell her how he feels.

Many men share Don's concern. While quite a few women have told me they feel very vulnerable when they express their ideas and are easily shamed by criticism or inattention, men are more likely to feel a certain amount of confidence when it comes to sharing their ideas, but feel vulnerable to feeling shame when they take the risk and express how they feel only to have their feelings ignored by an intimate or an audience. This makes sense. Middle class boys, on the average, are taught to expect others to appreciate their ideas and analytical prowess, but they are warned not to express their emotions too readily because doing so would not be manly. Girls, on the other hand, are taught not to be too intellectual—many are warned that would scare away potential suitors—but are encouraged to be open about their tender feelings. As a consequence, men tend to be more comfortable expressing their ideas while women are more confident about expressing feelings. There is nothing natural about this difference, it results from our gendered socialization, and it is always possible to change the way we raise boys and girls.

Don and I discuss the way boundaries were managed in his family: everyone was very proper, there was little spontaneity and less humor, and one did not talk about ugly, angry, embarrassing things. In his wife's family, her mother and sisters dominated, there were frequent emotional outbursts, and one had to learn to speak one's mind forcefully or risk never being heard. He wonders which kind of family is healthier. We talk about the difference in style between the two families, and the way that difference is reflected in the way he and his partner relate to each other. He imagines that if he had grown up in her family he would have expressed his feelings too timidly and then been mortified when his feelings were ignored. This perception helps him understand his wife's need to be so forthright in expressing her feelings. He decides to talk to her. Meanwhile—and this is entirely his idea—he will resist the urge to indulge in pornography: "It just serves to create distance between us so we never really talk about anything important."

The Aims of Therapy

Sometimes the therapist's task is to question the man's assumption that he must suppress aggression in his primary relationship. For Richard, the assumption derives from his feelings about the way his father treated him and his mother. The older man was a tyrant, ordering the family members around. When his mother failed to have dinner ready on time or said something wrong in front of company, his father screamed at her. Richard never saw his parents demonstrate much affection for each other, but he always assumed their sexual interactions were similar to their public displays—that is, his mother had to be available when his father wanted to make love, and he harangued her if she was not.

As an adolescent Mike was fairly passive with girls, and attentive to their needs. He was a good listener, and felt good when a girl told him she valued their friendship. But he did not have any sexual experiences. At his ten-year class reunion a quite attractive woman told him she had always had a crush on him in high school, but never told him so because she knew he was too shy to make any advances. This revelation led him to wonder why he had been so shy with girls during his teens, and he began to speculate that he was always trying very hard not to be a tyrant like his father. He bent over backward trying not to abuse women. They appreciated his sensitivity, but found him too passive.

In his relationship with his wife, he is still trying not to be a tyrant. He is not able to initiate sexual encounters for fear she will perceive him as too demanding, so he sulks when she does not approach him, and then eases the tension by resorting to pornography. We discuss the difference between an aggressive sexual advance and tyrannical abuse, and Mike begins to believe it might be possible to let his wife know he would like to make love without being a tyrant. Then, if she is interested they can proceed, if she is not there is no harm in his asking. Mike discovers something else about himself: When he distances himself from his wife and views pornographic videos he is unconsciously acting out a forbidden identification with his father. This leads to his exploring his relationship with his father, and making some distinctions there as well. His father was not always tyrannical, and there were parts of the older man that were well worth emulating. In fact, Mike could use a little more aggression in all of his pursuits. The trick is to figure out how to be aggressive without being abusive.

Don's mother was very intrusive and controlling while his father was emotionally absent and passive in relation to his mother, and a disappointing role model. Don remembers it being very hard for him to tell his mother to get out of his room or to stop talking to him so he could proceed with other activities, and he has similar difficulties telling his lover he is not interested in talking or doing something together. That is why he prefers living separately. He commits himself to be totally engrossed with her for the days they spend together, and then he totally detaches from her when they are apart. Pornography helps him enforce the boundary. In therapy he begins to see he can spend time with his lover while retaining some control of the boundary. For instance, after months of working on this issue, he reports that they are able to live together for a week at a time and he is able to spend some time alone and pursue his interests during that week. In addition, when they do return to their separate apartments, he feels less need to resort to pornography.

What lessons can be drawn from these cases? Of course, the sample is too small and the selection too skewed to warrant generalizations vis à vis the feminist debate on pornography. I have presented five examples of a special case: men who use pornography to cope with seemingly irresolvable relational dilemmas. From these cases we can assume that, for a certain number of men, pornography provides an escape from vexing aspects of primary relationships.

Is it better for a man to leave a relationship because he is sexually frustrated than to remain in the relationship and cope with his frustrations by resorting to pornography? Is it justifiable for men to objectify women in their imagination—that is, to create an imaginary sex life with pornographic women—in order to avoid mistreating the women with whom they relate intimately? These are difficult questions. It is not a therapist's place to judge. But in a certain number of cases I have found that the need to consume pornography is the obstacle men must surmount if they are to evolve a greater capacity for self-exploration and intimacy.

According to the antipornography movement, the consumption of pornography is wrong and men should be told to cease and desist immediately. But these men are already attempting to heed too many "oughts." In fact, their uncertainty and lack of vitality are caused by their attempts to satisfy all the oughts at once, especially when there seem to be contradictions between the oughts. Worse, in their attempt to escape from the contradictions they create a private space where they store a nonshared experience, and a new shame. A man in this situation begins to wonder if, when he gets to a place in a primary relationship where he and his partner are ready to do away with secrets, he will have to tell her about his pornographic experiences. The telling may not be a bad idea, but too many men, because they are frightened of such an eventuality, never permit intimacies to progress to the depth where they might be expected to disclose this kind of secret. The consulting room is a place where a man can risk new kinds of disclosure—and if nothing terrible (or judgmental) occurs there, a man can proceed to explore the pros and cons of making a comparable disclosure in a primary relationship, or with male friends.

If a therapist believes, as I do, that pornography is a symptom of a more pervasive malaise, one that affects all men in our society, then the question is not whether these men should be indulging in a sexist pursuit, rather, the question is how do we get there from here? Do we set up a set of oughts—for instance, it is wrong for a man to engage in private pornographic thoughts—and judge individuals harshly for their noncompliance; or do we understand pornography as a symptom and struggle to change what it is in an individual's psychological makeup and in our social arrangements that produces the symptom? In the very limited context of my consulting room encounters with sensitive men—I would not generalize these thoughts to the overt misogynist—I try to help men retrieve the parts of themselves that chronically hide out in secret places. Then, having reclaimed the passion that they had split off and left in those secret places, they are more likely to succeed in their struggle to create quality, nonsexist relationships.

CHAPTER SIX

The Conscientious Father and
the Unappreciative Son

Ihave seen several fathers in my office recently who were distraught over being rejected or physically or verbally assaulted by an almost grown or young adult son. These men take very seriously their responsibility as fathers. They were all caught off guard by their sons' attack or rejection, and felt hurt and unappreciated. The initial aim of therapy with these men is to understand why they react as they do to what they experience as a betrayal. Sometimes it is the son who seeks a therapist's counsel during a period when he is distainful and wants nothing to do with his father. The son needs to clarify for himself why he feels so compelled to distance his father. Of course, I do not see the father and the son unless both clearly desire family therapy. Instead, I tend to see the father from one family and the son from another. My clinical experience as well as my personal life as son and father lead me to witness, repeatedly, this curiously modern drama of the conscientious father and the unappreciative son.

In cases where the son was ignored or abused as a child and the father feels guilty about the way he raised his son, the son's rage seems appropriate enough and the negotiation is straightforward: the father feels remorse and asks the son's forgiveness; the son has the choice of forgiving or remaining furious. In cases where the father was neither absent nor abusive it is not as easy to understand the son's need to hurt and distance him. In fact, conscientious fathers do not understand where they went wrong and ask me to explain why their sons are acting so strangely. Meanwhile, the son does not quite understand why he is so disappointed and angry at his father—after all,

"Dad tried so hard to be a good father."

The two males are locked in a battle that does not make sense to either of them. Are they merely arguing about who is the greater disappointment?

The son's rebellion begins with disillusionment. The son attacks and devalues the father who disappoints. One can hope it is only a phase, but in cases where the father has been conscientious and does not feel blameworthy, it is not easy to convince the father to more or less patiently await a filial return. Instead, he becomes enraged. A father tells me his son pushed him against a wall, raised his fist menacingly, and then ran out of the house, not to be heard from in the intervening six months. He exclaims:

"How dare that little bastard treat me with such disrespect!"

I worry lest this father's rage mount to the point where he decides to cut his son off and never talk to him again. If the father burns all the bridges, the son runs a high risk of being stuck in a quagmire of disillusionment and resentment for life. I caution both fathers and sons that they should not make any permanent disconnection, they should permit themselves some rage about what has transpired, and perhaps take a vacation from each other, but neither should burn all the bridges. Time passes, as do the phases of adult life, including the phase wherein the young man needs to distance his father in order to get his own bearings on a life, and the phase wherein the older man feels a need to hold his son close before the two part ways and to give him that last little piece of advice.

Report of a Case of Father–Son Alienation

The son appears seeking help. He is twenty-one, halfway through college. He complains he is unable to focus his attention and complete his studies, and he is worried about his lack of interest in dating and sex. He tells me he has had no energy and has been losing weight for approximately six months, but he has only recognized his condition as a bout of depression for two months. His parents are divorced. He was twelve when they separated, and he spent his adolescence moving back and forth between their homes. His mother remarried, his father never did. His father established a very nice single-parent home. Father and son always remained close and loving, at least until six months ago. Then they had a fight—no blows, though it almost came to that at one point—and since then he has refused to speak to his father. He stopped visiting his father's home, and now when he returns to the area from his college in another locale, he stays at his mother's house. This really angers his father, he reports with a grin.

The son explains he is used to saying only things his father wants to hear, and now he suddenly finds himself criticizing and yelling at his father, usually over minor issues. His father does not receive criticism very well; in fact he takes it as a sign of disrespect, but the son has passed the point where he can act cordially and keep his anger from seeping out or exploding. So he refuses to speak, at least that way he tells no lies. Since he cannot refuse to speak in his father's presence—the older man believes silence is a sign of disrespect, too—he has decided to stop relating to him altogether. He realizes he has come to see me, an older male, in order to speak to someone like his father. I am his father's age.

"Perhaps," he tells me in a very somber voice, "if I can get you to understand what I'm going through I'll know I'm not entirely crazy to be this angry at my dad!"

With the son's consent I speak to his father. I discover that the older man spent his young adulthood as an activist in civil rights and antiwar movements and then became a very successful professional. He reports that he and his ex-wife went through the late 1960s together and, when the women's movement blossumed, struggled with each other to split housework and childrearing responsibilities equitably. He cut back at work while his son was very young. He prides himself on being unlike other men. For instance he was actively involved at the schools his son attended, often being the only father present at parents' meetings. After the divorce, he gave up a lucrative position in one city in order to follow his ex-wife and child when they moved to another locale. He is proud that he never lost contact with his son, but the move put his career in a tailspin and he is still not entirely happy with his professional accomplishments.

This father cannot understand his son's hostility toward him. He lists all he has done as a father and then asks if I think his son is being fair. He gave up career aspirations to stay close to his son, he runs a household on his own and provides well for his son, and he is forthright and flexible in this less-than-voluntary encounter with his son's psychiatrist. Later I ask the son if the father's list of his good qualities is accurate, and he says:

"Yes, my father was all those things. That's why it's so hard for me to hate him now!"

In other words, the father's "goodness," as well as the son's need to see the father in a positive light, makes it difficult for the son to express negative feelings toward the older man; but at some point all the unexpressed negative sentiments burst forth and the two do not have the kind of understanding between them that would permit such feelings to be explored openly.

The Son's Situation

As boys we believed that our powerful fathers would figure out a way to make the world safe for their beloved offspring. Our disillusionment came in stages. Heinz Kohut (1971) explains that some degree of disillusionment is inevitable every time a child reaches a new level of cognitive and psychological sophistication. Dad cannot remain Superman forever. Kohut worries about the sons who continue into adulthood idealizing their fathers. If the timing and dosage of the moments of disillusionment are right—and this means small, well-timed incremental disapppointments—the child develops ways to cope with disappointments and learns to accept the fact that all men are flawed to some extent, and still worthy of loving relationships. But if abrupt departures or disjunctions occur—the father abandons the family and fails to maintain contact with his son, or abuses the family, or lands in prison or commits suicide, or if the father desperately needs the son to continue idealizing him past the appropriate moment for disillusionment—then the son's psychological development suffers.

Peter Blos' (1984) explication of the stages of male development provides a context for understanding the son's disillusionment. He believes too little attention has been given to the negative Oedipus complex in males. The positive Oedipus complex is the boy's love for his mother and animosity toward his father. The negative complex centers on an early affectionate bond with father. According to Blos, it is not only the close relationship with mother that is internalized by very young children, an early loving bond with the father is also internalized and provides a "lifelong sense of safety in a Boschian world of horrors and dangers" (p. 303).

Blos believes that the boy's early positive bond with his father is repressed during the years when the positive Oedipus complex is played out; this is the time when incremental disappointments are likely to occur. The repression continues through early adolescence. This is the phase when the boy is busy developing exaggerated male characteristics in order to prove to himself and others that he is in fact a man. It is not until late adolescence that the negative complex surfaces again and the boy, by now confident that he is a male and is capable of loving a woman, can reaffirm his affection for his father. In fact, the boy must reaffirm this affection, or resolve the negative complex, if he is to progress to a healthy adulthood.

Blos' formulation sheds some light on the boy's crisis in late adolescence or early adulthood. In other words, in the ideal case the son has already expressed his negative feelings toward his father and is prepared for a reconciliation, but in many less-than-ideal cases the negative feelings surface late and make the son's leave-taking problematic. Often a nearly grown son complains that his father failed to prepare him to face the cruel world out there. Perhaps the father was overprotective, causing the son to feel unprepared when the time came for him to leave home. Perhaps the son feels that his father's ways do not work in today's world. There are many versions of the son's lament.

And the charge contains a kernel of truth, given the contemporary cultural context. American consumer culture is constructed on the assumption there will be qualitatively new styles and technologies every few years. These rapid stylistic and cultural turnovers cause people to feel that their three-year-old wardrobes, autos, compact disc players, and personal computers are outmoded. Meanwhile, consumers' distain for outdated styles and equipment creates a virtual bonanza for companies that depend on product obsolescence to expand their markets. In cultures that do not "advance" quite this fast, the wisdom of the elders is cherished and young men respect their fathers' opinions and utilize their fathers' wisdom in the conduct of their daily lives. But in American middle class culture, the advice of the elders seems off-target. Perhaps filial rebellion of some kind must eventually occur if the son is to become whole and independent and develop his own innovative ways of coping with a rapidly changing and increasingly hostile world.

In Lyle Kessler's (1983) play, *Orphans*, two orphaned brothers live alone until Harold, a nebulous gangster character, comes along to act as a surrogate father. Treat, the worldly brother who supports the duo with petty thievery had naive Phillip convinced he had to remain indoors all the time in order to avoid the "germs" that awaited him outside. Harold encourages Phillip to go outside in defiance of Treat's warnings, and Phillip nervously does so only to get lost in the big city. He retreats indoors, vowing never to go outside again. Then Harold gives him a street map, saying: "You're going to know exactly where you are in time and space." It is as if the father, who would soon be shot to death on the street, were saying to the son: "It's a dangerous world out there and I can't guarantee anyone's safety, so all I can give you is this map to help you navigate."

I am reminded of a dream I had when my sons were very young. I recorded it in my journal:

2/2/79: A Dream:

In sports arena-type building with Eric and Jesse (my two natural sons)—we are fighting with three men who have attacked us—One is my age, two are older—we run around the outside hall of a huge sports arena. I fight one man—beat him—run all around— find Jesse—help him fight his opponent—we run all the way around, anxious we can't find Eric—we finally find him—the three of us united beat up the third man.

My associations to the dream images: the hall is circular like my post-divorce apartment, in which the rooms are arranged around a staircase and a hallway encircles the staircase and provides a good place for a father to chase his sons—the older man is weak like my kids are in terms of street-fighting, like my father is, like I am—fighting vs. age—I want to be young to be with my kids—having kids is a way to fight the aging process. Circles: I run around in circles in my life. Mainly, the dream is about making the world safe for kids—trying to figure out how to raise them to have qualities I admire: sensitivity, creativity, openness, concern for others, unselfishness—but also the capacity to survive in a tough, competitive, cruel world. Will I be too old to help my sensitive boys cope with the world? Will the world be harder on them? Can I guarantee them a good future?

Some of the rebellion that precedes departure from the family home is a challenge to the father to step forward and make sense of it all for the conflicted son. If the father successfully arrives at the correct proportion of limit-setting and respect for the son's power—the former serving to help the son control his new-found powers, the latter to give him the message the father approves of his being powerful and independent—then the early affectionate tie can be renewed and strengthened, there can be a reconciliation, and the boy can leave home feeling both powerful and loved. This is the ideal scenario.

Robert Bly (1982, 1990) believes men—and he speaks mainly to men in their late thirties and older—must resolve leftover conflicts with their fathers if they are to be whole. Men need to acknowledge their fathers if they are satisfied with the way they were raised; if their fathering was not optimal they need to grieve for the father they never had and then make amends with the disappointing one who exists; or, if their father is dead, they can forgive him for his shortcomings and honor his memory. I think Bly's advice is very sound, if it is well-timed. Some men, even at midlife, have never gotten in touch with their anger toward and disappointment in their fathers; for them, forgiveness would be premature. But the suggestion that men grieve and forgive serves to short-circuit the kind of endless resentment that prevents men from moving on.

Sam Osherson (1986) interviewed adult men about their relationships with their fathers, and in presenting the results of his study includes many poignant stories from his own experience as a son and a father. He gives advice to men who would reconcile with their fathers, for instance: "One way of healing the wounded father is to plunge into your father's history. A man needs to find ways of empathizing with his father's pain" (p. 206). And he sums up with some good advice to the conscientious father as well as the unappreciative son:

> Healing the wounded father means accepting some of our aloneness, giving up the wish that Dad will take care of you, will set you on your feet so you'll never fear slipping. There is grief in that loss of the fantasied all-powerful father we wish we had. Accepting that loss means tolerating the wish for such a father and seeing that it is really a childhood dream. Our fathers harbored such a yearning too; it doesn't make one less of a man to admit to it. So one man could finally write of his father, "Dad, we share the same bewilderment, the same mystery in the face of what is." Seeing our fathers as human, accepting their frailties and lapses, allows us to accept our own frailties and imperfections in this world. (p. 212)

Philip Roth (1991) has written poignantly of his father's death from a tumor pressing on his brain stem. He comments:

> You can say that it doesn't mean much for a son to be tenderly protective of a father once the father is powerless and nearly destroyed. I can only reply that I felt as protective of his vulnerability (as an emotional family man vulnerable to family

friction, as a breadwinner vulnerable to financial uncertainty, as a rough-hewn son of Jewish immigrants vulnerable to social prejudice) when I was still at home and he was powerfully healthy and driving me crazy with advice that was useless . . . . (p. 180)

If the father is too invested in always looking good in the son's eyes, and the son, who is interested in pleasing the father, senses the father's need and continues to idealize him long after it is appropriate for a son to do so, then the moment of disillusionment may be postponed into early adulthood, and be quite traumatic. In the average developmental sequence there is a shift from idealization during the latency period—from age five until ten or eleven—to filial rivalry during adolescence (the positive Oedipal complex) and then to reconciliation during late adolescence (the reemergence of the negative complex). But the compliant son of a father who needs constant appreciation and praise for his fathering is likely to run into trouble when the disillusionments occur.

Prior to the time when the sons I am describing attacked their fathers or cut off contact, the sons' disillusionment had been an entirely private experience. This is the reason the fathers were caught off guard by their fall from grace. For instance, in those "happy families" where it seems to the outside world that everyone is having a good time, there are usually unspoken rules against criticizing one's father and openly expressing anger. R. D. Laing (1969) describes "happy families" where the members are required to act as if everyone loves each other and there are no significant conflicts, even if in actuality the children hate each other and feel abused or neglected by the parents. Laing's point is that the children are taught to pretend their family is something other than it is, and in the process they are alienated from their true selves. In such a family, when a rift in the filial relationship occurs, neither father nor son knows how to discuss the tensions in their relationship, and the son concludes they must separate.

The Father's Situation

A father whose twenty-four-year-old son refuses to have anything to do with him tells me he was not happy in his relationship with his own father; he continues to be disappointed in his father in various ways; and he would like to break the generational pattern and have a better relationship with his own son. To the best of this man's ability he has tried to be a different kind of father so his son would grow up without the emotional baggage he feels he is fated to carry, and he feels he has done a fairly decent job. He thinks he and his son have a good relationship—or at least he thought that until a few months ago. His son, who graduated college and moved to a city several hundred miles away, suddenly cut off contact with his parents, leaving them to wonder what they had done wrong.

There is another issue. Parents raise children with a vision of who the child will become. In the early years, the vision guides the parents' approach to the child, for instance: "You have to study if you want to go to college and get a rewarding job"; or "It would be nice if you expressed more appreciation to people who do nice things for you; they'll like you better and you'll have good friends." This is quite appropriate—to a point. Hans Loewald (1980) employs the parent's age-appropriate envisioning as a model for the therapeutic relationship:

> The parent ideally is in an empathic relationship of understanding the child's particular stage in development, yet ahead in his vision of the child's future and mediating this vision to the child in his dealing with him. This vision, informed by the parent's own experience and knowledge of growth and future, is, ideally, a more articulate and more integrated version of the core of being that the child presents to the parent. This 'more' that the parent sees and knows, he mediates to the child so that the child in identification with it can grow (p. 229).

At one moment of development the parent envisions and the child becomes. At another moment the child becomes someone the parent never envisioned, and the parent must step back from the role of child-shaper and begin to get to know and appreciate the unique and extraordinary child who is emerging. There are mini-crises in the progression, of course, when the child dresses outrageously, lies, breaks rules, stays out all night, experiments with drugs and sex, chooses friends whom the parents cannot accept, decides to drop out of school, and so forth. Sometimes it is the son's declared homosexuality that forces the parents to give up their preconceptions and either accept the unenvisioned offspring or risk losing him altogether. Stephen Levine (1992) captures the moment: "We hate them for not being who we hate ourselves for not being."

The son does best when the parents are willing to get to know anew a son who is unfamiliar in important regards, and one who they now know will never fulfill all their expectations. Sons can surprise fathers. The ones who seem a failure when they are in their early twenties can turn out to be real gems at age 30 or 40. The ones who seem to lack ambition at age 25 can turn around and get serious about their work at 30 or 35. Often it is the people who think the deepest about a variety of issues who take the longest to get started as adults. If one has to not only find a job that pays decently, but also must figure out whether the ethics of the company offering the job are acceptable—or the ethics of a whole profession—it takes longer to make decisions about what work to pursue. People who do not ask as many questions are able to get started on a career track sooner, but later they are more prone to unhappiness at work. I am generalizing, of course, and there are many exceptions.

The father is disillusioned when the son fails to become the man he had envisioned. If the father can cope, accept his son as an autonomous other, and let his son know he loves him for who he is, then the son is in a better position to accept himself in spite of his faults, to reconcile with the father who disappoints, and perhaps to become a father himself and pass the experience of constructive disillusionment on to still another generation. Sometimes it helps for the father to recall his own passage into adulthood, and consider the ways in which he was a disappointment to his father. Or the father might look into his own motives for wishing his son will turn out to be a certain kind of man—is he expecting his son to live out some of his unfulfilled aspirations?

A male client in his late twenties describes himself as a loser, "a n'er-do-well," and recalls that he never was able to satisfy his father's expectations.

"The old man wanted me to be a high-power lawyer, just like him. When I dropped out of college and started working in a cooperative produce market, he told me I'd never amount to anything. We didn't have much contact after that, until he got sick. Then it was too late. I went to see him a bunch of times before he died, but we never really talked. I've been moving around, living on subsistence wages. But it's hard to imagine myself ever really pursuing a career—I can't think of any that would make him proud of me, anyway."

In sharp contrast, another man, a gay professional in his mid-thirties whose father refused to talk to him for three years after he "came out" in his early twenties, tells me that his father has done an about-face. He lives in San Francisco, his parents in the East. Since their "reconciliation," he visits his parents on Christmas and Easter and they visit him at least twice a year. Recently he bought a new house with a long-term lover, and his parents came to visit. His father took him aside and said that he would have preferred for him to be doing this with a wife, but given his choice to be with a man, he was proud of his son's solidity and the way he and his partner were able to set up a warm and inviting home. During the same visit the father confided in the son that he was worried about his daughter, whose marriage was a lot less loving and stable than the son's long-term relationship. I do not mean this contrast to imply there is a causal link between the support a man receives from his father and his potential for success. Support helps, but it is far from a guarantee of success, and quite a few successful people suffered abuse or inattention as children.

My Own Experience

While still in elementary school I was out on an errand with my father when he nosed into a parking place just ahead of another car that was heading for the same space from the opposite direction. Before we could open the door a large man leapt out of the other car and approached our driver's side menacingly. He demanded my father get out of the car and fight. Dad muttered something about not having any reason to fight, and rolled up his window. The man slammed his palm on the fender, yelled at my father for another minute, threatened to break the window and haul him out of the car, and then turned, got back into his car, and drove away. Dad said very little, got out of the car, and ran his errand.

I was not shattered by this momentary disillusionment, and there were still many moments of disillusionment to come in our relationship. It would have been nice if we could have talked about the event. After all, I was struggling with the question of fighting or being called chicken, and here was my father "chickening out" of a fight. Did he think he was a chicken, or was he convinced, as I would become a dozen years later, that fighting whenever one is called out is a ridiculous thing to do? I did not talk with my father about all this and none of my friends talked with their dads about such things. In my early thirties I joined a men's group, and it was at one of the group meetings that I recalled some of my filial disillusionments.

Men's groups, like psychotherapy, provide a safe haven for taking risks, and often, when one is willing to expose a part of the inner life that had been painfully secret, great things can happen. Is it any surprise that so many men find that they end up talking in men's groups about their relationships with their fathers? As one member after another of my men's group talked about his father, I noticed that it was easier for the sons who had been severely abused to blow the whistle on their brutal fathers than it was for the sons who were treated pretty well to come up with a list of grievances. Lacking the venom, one is left to wonder what use there is in exposing all those embarrassing things about one's father.

One evening I took a deep breath and began telling my story: As a youngster, through my teens, I idealized my father and had little bad to say about him. I wanted to be like him, a physician who cared more about his patients than about making a profit—the model came from the novel, *The Last Angry Man*, which was made into a movie in my formative years. It was not until my third year of medical school that I realized that, though I loved the image of "the last angry man" battling the medical establishment, the actual practice of medicine held no appeal for me. That realization led me to my specializing in psychiatry so I could spend time talking to patients without having to be too concerned about their medical problems.

It was in early adulthood that I finally acted out my rebelliousness through radical politics. I should add that I do not believe it is fair to reduce social activism to unresolved Oedipal conflicts. It is, in almost every case, also based on a well-informed social analysis and sense of social responsibility, something we could use more of today (Kupers, 1993). And I cannot agree with those who selectively interpret activism as an acting out of unresolved Oedipal conflicts (Feuer, 1969; Bettelheim, 1971) while leaving the inactivism of the "silent majority" uninterpreted, as if it is normal to accept what is wrong with our social arrangements and abnormal to protest vigorously. But, in addition to being a time of righteous struggle for social justice, the 1960s were also a good time to do battle with one's father. I remember a meeting in a restaurant with my parents where they were arguing that my political activities were dangerous and would ruin my career. I was serving very publicly as the physician for the Black Panther Party and they worried lest I be arrested and my license be revoked. I countered self-righteously that their politics were neolithic, and that was why they were incapable of understanding the importance of my risk-taking. Things became quite heated and my father stormed out of the restaurant, leaving me to feel very pained by the fact that my principled political stance had to be a hardship for him.

I have been closer to my parents in recent years, but we rarely discuss our political differences. During the Persian Gulf War I was interviewed on radio in the city where my parents live. The topic was the mass psychology of war. They listened. A few days later I received a long letter from my father complimenting me on the eloquence of my argument against the war and the passion and sincerity of my commitment. Of course, he did not entirely agree with my position.

But he had obviously listened very closely, realized how my political stance was based on deeply held principles, and was able to let me know he respected my efforts to live by the principles I held dear. Until that exchange, while I knew in general that my father loved me and was proud of my accomplishments, I never knew if he really understood who I was; perhaps his love was based solely on the accidental fact that I was his son. Earlier I had told my men's group I wished my father would have known more about the person I was becoming and backed off earlier on giving advice about how I should live my life. The exchange about my radio interview finally made me feel recognized.

With my sons, I try to maintain closer communication than I had with my father. We have done a lot together. Still, there are moments when it is clear a son is disappointed in me. I teach a young son that he must follow the law and then I slow down when a police car appears and he tells me I am hypocritical, or I say something wrong in front of his friends and a slightly older son gives me a drop-dead look. Each son has serious complaints, too, and at a certain age he is very willing to tell me about them. For two of my sons the main complaint is that I divorced their mother when they were young. There are levels to their resentment about that, and we work through the issue as it resurfaces at each level. And sometimes the working through alternates with long periods of relative noncommunication, sometimes even mutual resentment. When I hear my sons' complaints I get a sinking feeling in my stomach and realize anew that I always wanted to believe I was a better father. Our children teach us humility.

From the 'Sixties to the 'Nineties

Each generation vows never to make the mistakes their fathers made. Perhaps it is a vow never to be absent, never to be abusive, never to fail to spend time teaching a son to throw a ball or understand a math problem. Each generation dreams of correcting all that was wrong with the parenting they received. The father's conscientiousness makes it very hard for him to accept the fact that his son might eventually be disillusioned with him and find him lacking in some very important regards, just as he found his father lacking. And the father is likely to feel hurt when the son expresses his disilluionment, and to feel unappreciated for all of his efforts to make things different for his son.

My father must have felt unappreciated, too; his idea of a good father was one who worked hard at the office and provided for the family better than his own father, a Jewish Russian immigrant who was barely able to provide for him and his brother and sisters. The fathers felt unappreciated when the sons rebelled in the 1960s; now the sons have grown up and feel unappreciated when their sons seem to be going off in yet a different direction.

What if I had come of age in a different decade and there had not been mass movements to provide a political rationale for jettisoning the ways of one's father? Perhaps I would have needed to distance myself from him in a different way, and then the distancing might have been as inexplicable to me as it is to the young men I see in my office today; and I might have felt as lonely in rebelling. Whereas, in the 1960s the son who rebelled against his father conceptualized his rebellion in political terms and had a large support network among counterculturalists and social activists, today's rebel is likely to be quite isolated. Like most other men, he lacks close male friends, and since he views his alienation from his father as a personal matter, he is unlikely to share his pain about it with anyone but a lover or a psychotherapist. The radical movements of the 1960s provided a slogan for filial alienation: "Don't trust anyone over thirty." In the absence of this kind of countercultural epithet today, many sons, as well as fathers, find themselves sitting in therapists' consulting rooms scratching their heads and wondering why it has to be this way.

The Male Theme

Freud explained how male concerns about dominance and hierarchy began. Borrowing from Darwin the notion of a primal horde, Freud (1913a, 1921) hypothesized that it was ruled by a jealous father who subjugated all the younger and weaker males and kept the most desirable females for himself. One day the sons banded together to kill and eat the father. (Freud, 1913a, traces cannibalism to this prehistoric event.) Then the brothers found that, lacking a tyrannical ruler to keep them in their place, they were prone to fight and kill each other as they competed for the women. Seeking to avoid constant bloodshed, they set up hierarchical religious and social institutions that henceforth would structure their social relations. They evolved a consensual authority structure so that they would not be compelled to fight constantly. According to Freud, our civilization was established in the interest of diminishing the ever present danger of intragroup and intergenerational violence. Of course, historians and anthropologists tend to disagree with Freud about the historical facts (Kroeber, 1920, 1939). Actually, Freud's story is a very nice piece of science fiction, but it does capture something about the male condition, and therefore contains an element of truth.

The male theme of topdog and fallen subordinate is passed on from generation to generation. Consider the case where the father has been anxious all of his life about the possibility he might fall to the bottom of the heap, and the son's most intense disappointment in his father occurs just at the moment of the father's fall. Arthur Miller explores this variation on the theme in *Death of a Salesman*, the denoument being every son's worst case scenario. There are other variations. The father who has worked very hard to reach the top may be disappointed in a son who is not ambitious, and even if the son decides to forgo the cutthroat battles that punctuate the climb to the top, there will be a scar in his psyche where his father's approval might have been. In fact, it is very difficult for young adults to manage financially today, even with a college degree. Many are deciding it is not worth it, or that they do not want to take part in the cutthroat competition in order to climb the ladder to success, and they are opting to live marginal lives or find low-paying jobs and live at home with their parents.

The manner in which the father copes or fails to cope with the male theme influences the son's options. One hopes that the father who has managed to attain a modicum of confidence in his own adequacy will be able to give his son—who is having a hard time making ends meet and deciding what career path to take—the message that he will love him no matter what he decides to do with his life. If the father feels secure enough to weather the moments of his son's intense disillusionment and somehow finds a way to maintain the continuity of the relationship in spite of the distance and animosity, the son is given the opportunity to work through his conflicted feelings toward his father while remaining confident that his father will survive and be flexible and understanding enough at a later time to permit reconciliation.

James Hillman (1964) conceives of the issue in terms of betrayal. According to him, in the early years, there is primal trust, the parent protects the child from his own treachery and ambivalence. But this situation "is not viable for life." Eventually the child is betrayed in the very same close relationship where primal trust is possible. In fact, according to Hillman:

> It may be expected that primal trust will be broken if relationships are to advance; and, moreover, that the primal trust will not just be grown out of. There will be a crisis, a break characterized by betrayal, which according to the tale is the sine qua non for the expulsion from Eden into the real world of human consciousness and responsibility (p. 7).

Hillman proceeds to a discussion of the father's "capacity to betray," an important ingredient in full fatherhood, and the son's related capacity to forgive.

Of course, the son's relationship with the father is not the only variable. Many men have been raised entirely by their mothers or by gay and lesbian couples, many have grown up in extended families and communes, and some men whose early interactions with their fathers were very traumatic have nevertheless become quite capable of quality intimacy. To focus for a moment on the son's interaction with the disillusioning father is not to say that the father is at fault for all the son's difficulties, nor that there is a single healthy model for family life.

Does it have to be as Freud predicted? Do men need hierarchical institutions in order to keep the peace, or might more cooperative and less hierarchical social relationships lead to a greater peace, and more justice? Alexander Mittscherlich (1969) examines the social consequences of this society's "fatherlessness," that is, the relative diminution of the father's status and power over the past century that has accompanied the process of industrialization and state intervention in family life. He believes there must be a strengthening of "conscious critical capacities" if society is to transcend the filial "omnipotence–impotence relationship" (that was characteristic of patriarchy) and make possible an "association between equals." The other possibility is that citizens will become frightened of the ensuing freedom and regress to patriarchal, hierarchical forms of social organization as German society did in the thirties. Mittscherlich's argument borrows from Erich Fromm's (1941) work and that of the Frankfurt School of critical theory (Jay, 1973).

I believe the choice we make as a society is related to the way fathers and sons handle disillusionment. The theme of disillusionment plays a big part in intergenerational strife. Even the overly idealizing son eventually becomes disillusioned in the father—and the way the father handles the moment influences the way the son is likely to handle disillusionment in the future. Too much disillusionment—or too much resignation in the face of disillusionment—can lead to depression or suicide. Or it can lead to total denial of the disillusioning reality and escape into fantasy and madness. The capacity to cope with disillusionment is an indispensable asset to a man who would live according to his principles in a very complex and constantly disillusioning world.

The drama of the conscientious father and the unappreciative son is repeated daily, even more so in this age of redefining masculinity. The drama can limit the redefining. If the father and son become frozen in their antagonistic stances, neither wanting to give in—as if both were transferring their training for success in the competitive business world to the filial competition—then both will suffer a great amount of pain and lose a valuable opportunity to reconcile.

Open discussion of these issues can be an immense help to father and son alike, even if the two discuss their relationship with their very separate support networks. But then male shame intrudes. Males who feel they are failing in the role expectations of father or son feel some shame and are consequently disinclined to share their pain with others and seek support. The result can be isolation. Alternatively, if the men can transcend shame and the impulse to isolate themselves, the support of others can help both father and son weather a period of alienation and begin to figure out ways to reconcile.

If the father is too inadequate, defensive, or rigid to permit the moment to pass and the reconciliation to proceed, then the son might develop very conflictual feelings toward powerful men. To the extent the male theme is involved in the filial dynamic, it helps if the father can figure out a third alternative stance vis à vis his son: if the father can see himself as neither topdog nor loser in the minidrama, then the son, too, might eventually learn to respect his father for the strong way he played his hand, and might be free to find a constructive third alternative for himself.

CHAPTER SEVEN

Men in Therapy

Psychotherapy occurs in a place apart. Freud invented the modern consulting room, a place where the rules of everyday life are suspended. It is not merely a matter of confidentiality, though that is important. There is also free association and a suspension of everyday politeness. The modern therapist modifies Freud's basic rule in asking the client to say whatever comes to mind. Men are encouraged to say what they cannot say anywhere else. In the world of men and work they cannot admit that they feel scared, confused, weak, or needy. They cannot say to their sexual partners that they fantasize sex with someone else or resort to pornography. In therapy they can try out new behaviors, for instance being vulnerable or getting angry at the therapist, and discover that the relationship will survive and even deepen in the process, unlike relationships they have had with a father, a partner, a colleague, or a friend.

A man can explore previously secret parts of his psyche, and enjoy being recognized as a larger human being by a therapist who has no interest in judging, prescribing, or converting him into someone other than who he is intent on becoming—or at least this is the ideal. Actually, psychotherapists vary in values and competence, and have their own hidden and unexamined agendas. But ideally, the consulting room is a place where a man can turn himself inside out and, when the pieces fall back into place, be a fuller person. Then the therapist and the client need to think about the man's reentry into a real world where the lessons of therapy must be applied.

More men are appearing in therapists' offices than ever before. After all, if a man has been successful enough to be able to afford psychotherapy, and he is feeling sufficient pain to override his disinclination to be dependent on another person, the rules of conduct in today's male culture permit him to consult a therapist when stresses overwhelm his capacity to cope, and usually there is no one else he feels free to talk to. And since the client pays the therapist to listen, the role of client is not entirely submissive; the therapist is on the client's payroll. Assured that no secrets will get out, and that he is not totally subservient, the male client can take an hour off from work, relax, and talk about the things he would never discuss with those who share his fast-paced, competitive life.

Some men immediately enter into power struggles with the therapist, some have a difficult time figuring out what to say and how to behave. I will discuss these two all too typical developments, describe a men's therapy group, and argue that friendship is an important issue to explore in therapy, particularly during the termination phase.

The Struggle for Power in the Consulting Room

Some men want to get right down to business and be done with therapy as soon as possible:

"I'm a very busy man. The only reason I've come is because I'm feeling so much anxiety lately that I've been unable to concentrate on my work. I'd like this to be a very short therapy—I can't really afford the time."

The therapy tends to be problem-oriented, and the man wants to end the therapy as soon as the crisis abates.

The power struggle might begin even prior to the first therapy session. Bill phones to set up an appointment to see me. His wife's psychotherapist recommended me. We try to find a time to meet. He wants me to make an evening time available. I tell him I do not have any evening times, and offer two or three times I do have open. He takes one. An hour before the appointed time his secretary phones to tell me he is too busy to get to the appointment, or even to the phone, and asks if I have an opening later in the day. I explain that my schedule is rather full, and offer a time later in the week. When that time arrives, he comes late and then is upset because I will not extend his session. Clearly the issue is not time, it is status. From his first call to make the appointment there were signs of a battle: Whose time is more important? Who is the more important man? Who is going to win this round and be able to set the time of our appointment?

Men size each other up. They learn to do it speedily. In the world of business, one risks being at a disadvantage if the other is not sized-up swiftly and accurately enough. Whether the other is a business rival, a potential friend or a therapist, there is always the fear of being defeated, dominated, or humiliated by him. The model is dominance and submission, the prevalent model for male relationships in our culture. If a man does not have a way to get the better of another man early in the relationship there is the danger of losing later.

Some men never get beyond this kind of sizing-up, not at work, not in their intimate relationships, and, sadly, not in therapy. They do undergo a certain amount of therapy, but only during crises, and they terminate as soon as they feel somewhat more in control of things. In other words, they are only willing to put themselves in a dependent position because their symptoms seem overwhelming, but as soon as their symptoms are partially alleviated their dread of dependency looms larger again and they leave. They may enter therapy after a particularly painful breakup of an important relationship, after a serious failure at work, because they are upset about the way a child is behaving, because they feel depressed and do not know the reason, or because they are experiencing a bout of impotence. Or their depression may follow a back injury or heart attack that forces them to slow their pace dramatically. Sometimes a man seeks a "quick fix" for his addiction to alcohol, drugs, gambling, or womanizing. And sometimes it is the occurrence of cancer or AIDS that brings a man to see a therapist. Most men hate feeling vulnerable and hate the idea of having to go see someone for help.

In therapy, men's traditional self-protective mechanisms get in their way. Afraid of dependency, they do not admit they are glad to have someone to talk to. Because they are afraid the therapist will think they are unmanly, they do not show their feelings or talk about their sexual difficulties. And because they learned very early never to trust another man, they keep the therapist at arm's length or entrap him in seemingly endless tangents.

Freud (1937) made this comment about such men:

> At no other point in one's analytic work does one suffer more from an oppressive feeling that all one's repeated efforts have been in vain, and from a suspicion that one has been "preaching to the winds," then when one is trying to persuade a woman to abandon her wish for a penis on the ground of its being unrealizable or when one is seeking to convince a man that a passive attitude to men does not always signify castration and that it is indispensable in

many relationships in life. The rebellious overcompensation of the male produces one of the strongest transference-resistances. He refuses to subject himself to a father-substitute or to feel indebted to him for anything, and consequently he refuses to accept his recovery from the doctor (p. 252).

Object relations theory attributes this characteristic power struggle to the expression of a narcissistic trait, a trait shared by a large number of men. Kernberg (1975) insists the therapist must confront and interpret the anger that lies behind the client's need to seize power in the consulting room, whereas Kohut (1971) encourages the therapist to empathize with the pain and hurt that underlie the anger. On the one hand, the man devalues the male therapist in order to feel superior (meanwhile despairing of ever finding a father substitute powerful enough to help him); on the other hand, he wishes the therapist will prove to be quite powerful but worries lest his envy of such a powerful man get out of control. The therapist must avoid choosing either horn of the man's dilemma, and must find or create an opportunity to talk to the client about this pattern in his relationships. Perhaps during a course of therapy the psychological roots of the man's need to both devalue and idealize other men can be uncovered, and the client can overcome the ambivalence that prevents him from feeling close to others.

The therapist must figure out a way to connect with the man, to gain his trust. The dominance/submission issue figures prominently. I felt I must not act too submissively with Bill, for instance giving in and creating an evening hour for him, lest he judge me a pushover and decide that no man as weak as I seem to be could ever help him with his problems. (Of course, if I happen to have an evening hour open, why be inflexible?—his conflicts about power will show up again in another context.) But I knew if I did not accommodate his bid for power, he would feel too small and intimidated in my presence to trust me and open up.

Another client, Arnold, had to get past that hurdle before he could derive any benefit from psychotherapy. At first he was uncomfortable in my office. He coped with his anxiety by being very intellectual. He cited scholarly references in the middle of making a point. He would pick apart the comments and interpretations I offered. I became defensive. Feeling battered, I began to stand up to him a little more. At one point I even insisted that an interpretation was correct, and that he was denying it. He arrived for the next session stewing. He said he was very disappointed in me, losing my cool and attacking him as I had done in the previous session.

I was taken aback. I had not felt that the last session had ended badly. We had eventually arrived at a revised interpretation that we both agreed fit his situation, explored some of the reasons he needed to deny the validity of my interpretations, and the session had ended on a warm note. Now he was clearly angry at me. He felt he had reason to be:

"It was your insensitivity. I was very hurt by your accusation that I purposely deny the validity of your interpretations. It's hard for me to be talking to a therapist. I'm being as open as I can with you, I'm trying as hard as I can to share my feelings. Maybe I have to put up an intellectual smokescreen occasionally, but you're a therapist and you should know that's just to cover up my nervousness."

During the first phase of this man's therapy I repeatedly found myself fluctuating between a feeling I had to stand up to him or be seen as too weak to help, and the feeling that I had to be more gentle, more empathic, and more responsive to his pain and vulnerability.

The negotiation around scheduling offers an opportunity to talk about conflicts men have about engaging each other on an intimate level, and the problems the client has coming to another man for help. It is the accuracy and relevance of the therapist's comments and interpretations that convince the man that this therapist has sufficient power to help him with his problems, but it is the therapist's empathy, warmth, and his willingness to respect the client's defenses and slow the pace of interpretations that permit the client to trust the therapist enough to open up a little more about his conflicts and fears.

Rudy arrived for his first appointment fifteen minutes late. He had been laid off from a very prestigious and lucrative job, and he was depressed. The layoff shattered his image of himself as a star: a star athlete and student body president as a youth, a star businessman as an adult. He became depressed and impotent. He was unable to face his friends, much less talk to them about his feelings. He was not even able to ask them to serve as references on job applications. And he was so depressed he could not imagine interviewing for a new job—he feared his depression would be obvious and he would be rejected. We began a course of psychotherapy. No time was designated. I shared my understanding of our agreement as of the end of our first session:

"We will get started, we'll see what we uncover and what improvements result, and then we'll talk again about how long we should go on meeting."

His depression lifted after four or five weeks. He failed to appear for our sixth session. I phoned. He told me that he was feeling better and would not need to come to see me anymore. In fact, he had found a job a few days prior to the missed session, and merely forgot to call and cancel. I said I was happy about his good fortune, adding that I would have felt better if he had called and cancelled. In fact, I told him, I thought it would be a good idea for him to come in for one more session where we might have the opportunity to talk about ending this therapeutic relationship; I would feel better about parting, and my guess is he would too. He agreed. Rudy began the session with an apology for having "hung me up." I asked:

"What was that all about?"

"I guess I just got so excited about getting the job, and I had to get busy getting ready to work, I guess I just forgot about the appointment."

"That explains your not cancelling. But I wonder if there isn't more to discuss about the incident. For instance, could it also be that you're not real happy about having to be in therapy, and you're anxious to get it over with? And isn't it pretty tough to say goodbye in person?"

He agreed on both counts. I suggested that he might gain something from spending a little time talking about why it is so hard for him to say goodbye in person. He admitted the pattern is familiar, for instance he repeatedly finds himself ending a relationship with a lover by just never seeing or calling her any more. He wonders out loud whether it might be better to call a woman up and talk about ending the relationship. He thanks me for making that connection between the ending of this therapy and the ending of his romantic relationships. In fact, he continues, he really appreciates all the insights I've shared with him.

"You should know this short therapy has done me a lot of good. I think you must be pretty good at what you do."

He confesses his sadness about our parting. I tell him I am sad about our parting too, and leave the door open for him to return to see me as needed.

Sometimes, when it is clear the new client alternates between idealizing and devaluing the therapist, it helps to tell him that he might feel like leaving after a few sessions when he feels a little better. Then, when the client does begin to feel better and thinks of terminating therapy precipitously, he will remember that the therapist predicted this might happen. The prediction serves two purposes: The client might be impressed with the accuracy of the prediction and begin to value the therapist's interventions more; and the prediction creates a bind for the client who is intent on proving the therapist wrong—if he does terminate precipitously the therapist was correct in his prediction. This might cause him to reconsider terminating, at least long enough to discuss the issue with the therapist. Arnold Goldberg (1973) outlines a useful strategy for therapists working briefly with men who suffer from what he terms "narcissistic injuries," the first step being to empathize with the man and support his faltering self-esteem. Only after a modicum of self-esteem is restored will he be able to listen to interpretations.

Problems Filling Emotional Space

There is another kind of male therapy consumer. Instead of swaggering and trying to take over like the men I have described, these men tend to be shy and uncomfortable in a therapist's office. They admit they do not quite know why they have come and ask for a lot of directions from the therapist about how they should act.

One man explains: "It's better if you ask the questions, I've never done this kind of thing before, I wouldn't know what to talk about."

Another tells me: "You're the expert. I want to figure out how to tell you what you need to know to get me patched up. If I just ramble we'll never get to what you need to know."

They also cannot say with much conviction how they are feeling, and complain they do not really know their true desires. For many of these men it is a matter of taking care of others' feelings so much that they are out of touch with their own. These men do not operate on the premise that when one man sets foot in another's office a battle for power must ensue. They are more interested in pleasing the therapist than they are in battling for power.

Are they merely laying down on their backs and saying they give up, that the therapist is boss? Are they surrendering to the Oedipal father? Or are they too mature, too well-grounded to engage in battles with me? Are they assuming they should follow my lead if they want my help? Or do they have little or nothing to say? Maybe they are so out of touch with their feelings and so unpracticed in talking about what is on their minds that they simply cannot speak extemporaneously to a therapist. In any case, the contrast between these men and the ones I first described makes one wonder if the second group is not just bending over backward to be certain they do not appear as narcissistic as the first group.

There is a flatness among these men. They have great difficulty filling emotional space in the consulting room, just as they do in their everyday lives. They do not initiate conversations or express feelings. They do not speak of inner events in the time we have together. Most importantly, they lack vitality and spontaneity, and seem unaware they have some responsibility for keeping our encounter alive. These men are not simply depressed. One can talk about depression in a dead way or with a certain amount of aliveness; one can slump in the chair and speak in monosyllables or one can gesture with one's arms and sob. Of course, depression plays a part in each man's story. But there is something here about gender, too. Men tend to have difficulty filling emotional space.

There are a number of explanations of a man's inability to fill space in an interpersonal encounter. Eva Seligman (1982) calls these men the "half-alive ones," and suggests that their lack of vitality is a result of their childhood experience in a family with an emotionally absent parent, usually the father. Sean Cathie (1987) believes the man's passivity and lifelessness arise from an overidentification with his mother and a lack of sensitive male role models. Richard Meth (1990) argues that men are devoid of feelings because they are encouraged to express only what is permissible according to the rules of traditional masculinity and to avoid behaving in feminine ways, and this means they are conditioned not to express feelings.

Heinz Kohut (1971) feels these men suffer from a "disorder of the self," expressed as "insufficient narcissistic libido." Essentially, Kohut believes that a certain amount of attention—for instance, parents clapping or beaming when a child takes a first step or says his first word—is required for an individual to develop the sense that he or she has something to offer that deserves attention or applause. If parents were too narcissistic themselves to provide enough empathy and attention at certain critical moments, then the child grows up with a disordered sense of self and an inability to express himself with any animation and force.

Alice Miller (1981) describes people who, from infancy, learn that their parents cannot consistently care for them, and that, in order to feel connected to such narcissistic parents, they must in effect take care of their parents. As adults, such people tend to be better at taking care of others than they are at expressing their own feelings, desires, and needs. Men who fit this pattern tend to take care of their partners very well, but rarely demand attention to their own needs, and on account of this tendency become depressed.

There are many explanations for men's difficulties in filling personal space and space in the consulting room. As I explained in

Chapter One, I believe that many of these men are trying so hard not to be brutish that they have difficulty doing or expressing anything very forcefully. Of course, all of these explanations of men's lack of vitality are additive. When a child lacks a sensitive role model, is the recipient of little or no applause for his early achievements, grows up thinking his job is to take care of others, and wants to avoid being a brute and putting himself forward too forcefully, he is predisposed to develop into a man who is incapable of filling emotional space.

What about male clients with women therapists? Helen Meyers (1986) believes that the gender of the the therapist does affect the treatment, "but only in terms of the sequence, intensity, and inescapability of certain transference paradigms in therapy" (p. 263). Michele Bograd (1990) describes some of her experiences treating men, including her feeling intimidated by men's anger and feeling she should be the one to fill the void between the two participants. She relates these themes to the reality of domination and gender inequity in our society. Teresa Bernardez (1982) explains how women can utilize traditional female capacities to aide their therapies with men. For instance, the woman can begin with tenderness and openness as the man begins to share his feelings, she can give him permission to openly grieve, and she can tolerate the love he feels in the transference as well as the rage he displays when he feels rebuked. I find I learn quite a bit about men in therapy by reading the reports of women therapists, but there are also differences when men treat men.

One strategy I find useful with men who are unable to fill emotional space is to look for moments of real aliveness in the therapeutic encounter and then ask why there are not more moments like that. For instance, when one male client begins to talk about his parents and his early childhood, I am quickly bored by the deadpan presentation of facts. He mentions a fishing trip he went on with his father, his face seems to light up, and there is more intonation in his voice. Then he returns to the chronology of childhood events and his voice becomes flat again. I comment about the momentary sign of liveliness and he tells me the fishing trip was a wonderful event. I ask why he said so little about it, in spite of the fact it seemed to be the part of the story he was most excited about, and he says:

"I thought I was supposed to tell you all about my past. If I say more about the fishing trip we'll never get done with the whole story by the end of the session."

In other words, this man thinks that completing the story is more important than selecting a part that is compelling for some reason.

Since I never asked him to talk about anything in particular, I ask where he got the idea he should complete his chronology.

He responds: "I thought that's what you're supposed to do in therapy."

Next we talk about the difference between talking about what one is "supposed to" talk about, and choosing one's own agenda with a therapist or with anyone else.

He says: "I guess I'm not very good at knowing what I want to talk about."

I ask if this might explain the flatness in his voice. He gets the point and decides to continue talking about going fishing with his father. Meanwhile, his voice and gestures seem more animated.

Another male client admits that he tones himself down in various situations, especially in the company of men, because he fears that a display of his enthusiasm and wit might threaten other men, or make them envious, and then they might attack him. If therapy is successful, the male client learns to stay in touch with feelings and desires, and no longer needs to grimace uncomfortably and hunt frantically for words when asked how he is or what he would like to do or talk about.

A Therapeutic Men's Group

A few years ago, as I sat in my consulting room listening to one man after another flatly and matter-of-factly relate his story, I decided to try to bring these men together in a group. Many of the issues these men brought to therapy were related to conflicts around being a man. I thought it would be worthwhile to talk about them in a group. I had been in a leaderless men's group for several years and learned first hand about the ambivalencies surrounding modern manhood. I felt I could share some of what I had learned, and perhaps help a group of men connect and relate in new and meaningful ways (Gordon & Pasick, 1990; Solomon & Levy, 1982; Sternbach, 1990).

I invited most of the fifteen men I was then seeing in therapy to join the group. Less than half opted to do so and one could assume that those that did tended to be more willing to admit their dependency feelings. Two gay clients declined, saying they did not want to be put in the role of instructing straight men on how to be intimate with other men.

During the early group sessions the group had difficulty filling emotional space. It seemed to have trouble getting started, both at the beginning of sessions and whenever a member's issue had been discussed for awhile and it became obvious it was time to move on. I could tell from the glances directed my way that the men were being less than spontaneous out of concern about my approval, a dependency issue that must be addressed periodically in any therapy group. We discussed concerns about any one of them "hogging the floor," and fears that without me to lead and control the discussion, petty squabbles would erupt. I thought more about why the feeling of emptiness prevailed and I eventually asked:

"Why is it so hard for anyone to think of something to say next?"

The response sounded straightforward:

"It just isn't easy."

After some discussion, everyone agreed it was something about being men and the group discovered a shared pattern among several who are married or in long-term committed relationships: Each man relies on his partner to a great extent to supply the "juice" between them. Without the partner present, these men lack knowledge, drive, or passion to produce the juice. How can a bunch of men who are all dependent on women to make them feel fully alive hope to generate any emotional life in a group therapy setting with a relatively silent therapist?

I notice that each time a group member raises a personal dilemma, the group talks about the man's problem for awhile and then begins to repeat itself as if no one knows how to attain closure on one topic and move on to the next. I step in a couple of times, ask the man who presented his dilemma if he has gotten what he wants from the discussion, and when he says he has I ask who else wants to share a dilemma. The third time this pattern is repeated I elect to remain silent, and the group perseverates on one member's dilemma. I ask what is going on. The men eventually arrive at the conclusion they are all hesitant to interrupt a discussion of one man's issue in order to raise their own. They are aware of an urge to interrupt, but they repeatedly decide that would be rude, and they do not want to act too aggressively in the group. I ask why not and we proceed to a discussion of their fear of violence erupting in the group.

"So," I introject sharply, "the group's fear of rivalry and violence causes a certain deadness in the room!"

They agree, and one says that in mixed groups he usually leaves it to the women to shift the topic of conversation:

"They seem to be able to do that without anyone getting too upset about being cut off."

What I see in the consulting room raises questions regarding men's ways of relating. Can men construct with each other a relatedness which is compelling, safe, and allows them to draw energy away from their lives with women? This is an important question for many reasons, one being that couples are finding that the quality of their primary intimacies is better when both have close friends. And if the woman has close friends while the man does not, the inequity can create serious tensions in the primary relationship. In Chapters Seven and Ten I will discuss the importance of same-sex intimacies in the struggle to change gender roles and gender relations.

In a therapy group, where the task is to understand oneself and one's interactions with others, and the leader does not structure the process to any great extent, there are awkward silences. Unless the men change, the group seems doomed to stiffness and boredom. These men do talk to other men—usually at work, or about a particular topic, or while sharing an activity such as watching or participating in sports events. They usually have no trouble filling space with task-related talk in those contexts. And this is very important. Too often men are criticized for relating only while doing a project or watching a football game. But this kind of shared activity can be the basis for a deeper connectedness between men. Many men report that the man they go to for support when they are in dire need, and the man with whom they feel free to cry, is the man with whom they once survived a frightening ordeal or teamed up with to win an important athletic contest. The problem arises when men fail to move on to deeper levels of intimacy and the mindless doing and watching together becomes the totality of male relatedness.

In the therapy group, the discussion immediately takes off if I give each man a task. When I suggest that each group member spend a few minutes talking about his relationship with his father the anxiety level in the room diminishes. Each man suddenly knows what is expected of him and the members take turns, each giving an orderly if somewhat cursory description of his relationship with his father. It inevitably becomes an emotional event. Someone breaks down and cries, giving others license, or someone discovers a similarity between his experience and that of another member, and feels reassured by the similarity.

During one session a group member shared with the others a very embarrassing problem he was having. At the very last minute of the group session, for a number of weeks, Joe said he had something important to talk about, something that was keeping him from asking a woman out on a date. For several weeks following the first announcement the group forgot to return to this man's important issue, and he was too timid to mention it again until the final minute. Finally, at the beginning of one group session, one of the members expressed a desire to hear about the important issue.

Joe's face turned crimson, but he was able to blurt out a description of a sexual problem. The men, by this time feeling very close and trusting with one another, were sensitive both to this group member's dilemma and to his embarassment talking about it. A few of the others admitted that they too had experienced sexual difficulties. Someone then suggested that Joe might find it helpful to talk about his problem with a woman, that is, when he meets a woman with whom he feels close enough to be sexual. Joe resolved, in front of the group, to implement the suggestion as soon as he met a woman he liked.

A week later Joe risked asking a woman out on a date for the first time since the sexual problem arose six months earlier. At its next session the group discussed the fact that he had exposed himself to potential humiliation, and was dependent on the group for a sympathetic response if he was to sustain his fragile sense of manliness. But he did take the risk, and permitted himself to be vulnerable for a moment. And other group members said they felt very good about the fact he was able to trust them. Discussion turned to the way men feel they always have to be in control, and how hard it is to permit oneself to be vulnerable or dependent. In the weeks that followed the upbeat conclusion to this episode, several men commented that they found themselves thinking about this group experience, and wishing they could have had discussions like that with their fathers. As the discussion proceeded past the moment when tears became evident in the eyes of several members, I noticed that the group seemed more consistently vital, the problem filling space having disappeared for the moment. Several members of the group reported that, in their lives outside the group, they were taking more risks of the kind Joe had taken, and were finding that they felt closer to the people with whom they were taking the risks.

Friendship and the Termination of Therapy

After the original crisis that propelled a man toward therapy is close to being resolved, he often discovers other reasons for seeking help. Perhaps he also very much wanted to discover how to feel more alive, how to play and have fun, or how to bring vitality into his intimate relationships. It is more difficult for men to admit that they would like to be able to have friends again, close buddies like the ones they had in high school or college. Typically, after the acute symptoms subside, men are faced with a choice about continuing therapy. The man can continue in therapy and probe deeper, hoping to change more longstanding patterns. Or he can terminate this therapy and return at a later date if he feels the need. Or he might want to enter a men's group, with or without a therapist as group leader.

John remained in therapy nearly three years. He attended semi-regularly. He cancelled an average of one out of three or four weekly sessions. Each time he entered the consulting room he apologized for having to be here again, seemed a little perplexed about why he continued to see me, and proceeded to explain a problem that was troubling him in his marriage, with his children, or at work. Typically we put our heads together and solved the problem, or at least found a next step to solving it, and explored some of the psychological conflicts that made the problem seem so familiar. Sometimes we talked about his wish that his father would have spent this kind of time problem-solving with him. His father had always been too busy. John would stop just short of saying he appreciated my efforts.

In the middle of a scheduled three-week break in our sessions John called to say he would not be able to come to our next appointment. The message contained no return phone number and he said he would call when he was ready to reschedule. That seemed an instruction not to call, so I heeded it. Two weeks later I received a lovely note from John in which he thanked me for being so helpful and told me he felt the therapy had accomplished quite a bit. He felt changed in some ways, which he briefly described. And he said his ambivalence about dependency remained, and he was choosing to sever our therapeutic relationship for now and this was the only way he felt comfortable doing so. I honored his request and did not phone or write.

Other terminations proceed in more orderly fashion. I have written extensively about the termination phase of therapy (Kupers, 1988.) Here I will address one issue that comes up during the termination phase, a crucial one for men: friendship. Friendship is problematic for the average man. He has many "buddies," guys with whom he works, plays sports or "hangs out." But he has few if any male friends with whom he can share his emotional life. The average middle class white male is more likely to share his personal experience with women: a wife or long-term partner or women friends whom he finds more trustworthy and more "there" than any of his male buddies. This was a theme in the therapy group. Men usually discover that they like talking with a therapist about their inner lives. Whereas the men in the group can practice new ways of relating with each other during sessions, men in individual therapy have to find men in their everyday lives if they are to put into practice what they learn in therapy about feeling more connected and alive in their relationships.

Many men enter therapy during a crisis in a primary relationship. If a man's female partner is his main or only confidante, and she becomes furious with him during a stormy period in their relationship, he is left with no one to talk to about his situation. So he goes to see a therapist. The therapist becomes his sole confidante. If, during the course of therapy—as one hopes—the relational crisis is resolved, the couple is once more on speaking terms. Then, with his partner in his corner again, the man chooses to terminate psychotherapy. What, I usually ask him, will happen the next time he and his partner get into a fight?

Men admit they have few real friends. And they do not understand why. There are the oft-cited theoretical causes—homophobia and societally induced competition and distrust of other men—but on a personal level, men have a hard time explaining why they have never succeeded at maintaining close male friendships. I have explored two patterns in therapies where both participants are men: a continual battle for dominance, and a problem filling emotional space. These two patterns also crop up in men's same-sex relationships outside of therapy. Perhaps the lessons of therapy can be usefully applied to friendship. By controlling power struggles and exploring their roots and then building on the moments of real vitality that do occur in the consulting room, perhaps men can learn to deepen their same-sex intimacies.

If a man wants to explore this in psychotherapy, the therapist can be a great help, especially as termination nears. The therapist asks the obvious question: Who will replace me as the sole confidante outside your primary relationship? Of course, there are important differences between a therapeutic relationship and a friendship, but to the extent the therapist's presence in a man's life satisfies certain here-and-now needs for intimacy, the client must work on finding others to fill those needs. In other words, an examination of the client's network of intimacies might usefully be part of the agenda for therapy during its termination phase. The therapist can help the client get started building the network of intimacies that will make the therapist's absence from that network tolerable for the client. I am convinced that until that task is accomplished, the client is not fully prepared to terminate. Since friendship is such an important issue for men, I will devote the next chapter to its exploration.

CHAPTER EIGHT

Friends

About a year ago I had a huge fight with a good friend, and an opportunity presented itself to reverse some of my old patterns. We had been friends for many years. His female partner told him some angry things about me. I was hurt by her disdain. I asked my friend whether he felt the things she said about me were true. He seemed uncomfortable with the question and took several minutes to answer. Then he said he had thought about it, and no, he did not think her castigation of me matched the reality very well. Then, I demanded to know why he did not defend me in discussions with his partner. Why did he not tell her he disagreed with her negative assessment of me? It was a calm, reasonable discussion. He thought about what I was saying and we parted on good terms.

We did not talk for a few weeks, leaving each other messages about arrangements to get together for lunch. I had to cancel one date because of a son's illness. When we finally did make phone contact, he informed me he was angry at me for always cancelling dates. I responded sharply that I was angry that he had so little concern about my sick child, and so little understanding of how difficult it was for me to arrange to meet him for lunch, considering my responsibilities at work and at home. We argued, we yelled at each other, and I slammed the phone down. My wife and son were surprised to hear me yelling on the phone, but when they realized who I was yelling at they began to cheer me on—it seems they had always been critical of my "How-are-you-fine-and-you?" style of relating to men friends. My friend and I talked again a few days later, and patched things up. In fact, the spontaneous emotional outburst seemed to clear the air between us and permit a little more spontaneity in our relationship.

I have close friends, and we can be quite intimate, but I have to admit that my relationships with friends could be vastly improved. What brings this point home is a tendency to compare my intimacies with those of my wife, who, quite frankly, prioritizes friendship higher than I do. For instance, when we arrive home from a family vacation, as soon as the car is unpacked and our sons are off to their rooms or their friends' houses, Arlene goes to the phone to share some of her vacation stories with two or three friends while I, feeling slightly relieved the phone is tied up so I will not be disturbed, head for my computer to get on disk some of the ideas that were germinating while we were travelling.

Besides the four or five couples that my wife and I see often, I have approximately a half dozen male friends with whom I have lunch regularly, perhaps once or twice a month. Since I try to be home with my family for dinner, weekends are usually busy, and I am tired in the evening after a long day at work, lunches are the best time to see friends. The lunch meetings are generally quite enjoyable, and there is talk of intimate things. But, at the same time, there is a certain lack of spontaneity. After all, the most compelling events in my life occur sporadically, and not always just prior to a scheduled lunch meeting with a particular friend. Thus, on the average, when asked by one of these friends how I am, I must scan memories of the past week's events in order to select a fitting subject for discussion. Sometimes I end up giving a very coherent summary of events and relationships, a summary that lacks the immediacy that would accompany the telling if I happened to be talking to this particular friend at a moment of confusion, anxiety, or sadness.

And why don't I pick up the phone and call a friend at such times? Partly it is because my wife is readily available, and like most of my male friends I reach out first to the woman who occupies a central role in my life. Partly, I tell myself, it is because I hate talking on the phone. I used to think my distaste was idiosyncratic, an aftereffect of having been on call too much as a young physician and dreading the phone's ring. Then I read Lillian Rubin's (1985) report that most of the men she interviewed shun speaking on the phone. Most of my male friends and clients avoid telephone conversations. Is it the phone that men dislike, or the immediacy of another man's presence at times of need and desire? Isn't the phone merely an instrument that might permit us to have immediate access to a male friend if we really wished it? I do not believe most women like the phone (the instrument) as much as they like the immediacy of the contact—the availability of a friend at a moment when the feelings are at their peak. I prefer to wait until the emotions abate. I tend to retreat from my friends when I am most acutely troubled, and tell them of my troubles only in retrospect, after I have restored my grip on things. Perhaps this is why my lunch meetings with friends seem somewhat flat. Of course, part of the difficulty I have being friends with men is an idiosyncratic expression of my personal foibles and part is related to gender.

Isaac Bashevis Singer (1962) tells the story of a group of friends he had as a youth in the Jewish ghetto in Warsaw. He was the leader. One day he decided the others resented him and were excluding him from their conversations. He wondered if he "had sinned against them, or deceived them. But if so, why hadn't they told me what was wrong?" He decided to wait it out. Contact between him and his friends was broken off and he pursued his studies, alone. Time passed. Singer tells of the attempt of one friend to approach him and try to persuade him to make the first move toward reconciliation. He refused: "I was infuriated. 'It wasn't I who started this,' I said. 'Why should I be the one to make up?' " Eventually his friends sent him a note saying they missed him. They confessed they had been wrong and begged his forgiveness. He became the leader again, and delighted them by reading the stories he had written while estranged from them.

As a therapist, I see many men who lack friends, or wish they had more close ones. For instance, a client tells me he thinks he is boring me, and that is why I yawn during the session. He wonders whether the reason he has no close friends is that men find him boring. This leads to a discussion about the line between his personal issues—for instance, the way his lack of connection with a depressed and distant father ill-prepared him to trust his ability to inject vitality into his relationships with other men—and men's difficulty, as a gender, "filling emotional space" in their same-sex relationships. As I mentioned in Chapter Seven, the process of therapy eventually leads to an exploration of one's circle of intimates, and each client reports his own reasons to be wary of close male relationships. In most cases, men do not visit therapists seeking help with their friendships. But while the therapist and client search for the meanings that lie behind the symptoms, the subject of friendship comes up, or if it does not come up by the time of termination, I bring it up.

A Clinical Vignette: Sean

Sean, a business executive in his mid-forties, suffers from panic attacks—intense palpitations and sweating that break out suddenly and without warning, often causing him embarassment at the office and at dinner parties. He has a wife and child and lives in a relatively affluent neighborhood. His company is big, a point he stresses in our first therapy session. He tells me he has been depressed lately, and not sleeping. He is experiencing daily bouts of panic. He is not quite sure what is bothering him, but he knows he cannot remain this depressed and panicky much longer and continue functioning at work.

During the first few sessions we review the areas of his life where there might be a problem. He tells me he is unhappy at work; they have passed him over for a promotion and he feels his future in the corporation is very uncertain. He is having an affair, and explains that his wife gives him little sense of himself as a virile, desirable man. And his teenage daughter hates him—

"She thinks I'm more interested in work than in her and, you know, there's some truth in that."

I ask Sean whom does he talk to about his problems, and he tells me there is no one he can trust; that is why he has come to see me. He cannot talk to colleagues. They are either superiors who might hold him back if he reveals to them his personal problems, peers who might use what he tells them to get ahead of him in the office, or subordinates with whom he feels he must maintain the image of somene who "has it all together." And he cannot seem to find the time to get together with friends outside the work setting. In other words, he has no friends. In fact, he realizes as we begin to discuss the subject, part of the reason he began the affair was that he felt he could no longer talk to his wife about his feelings and sought out the comfort of sharing his thoughts with another woman.

We discuss Sean's concerns in turn, and begin to make some headway. During one session Sean mentions a fleeting thought that I might be recording our conversations, and quickly shifts to another topic. I ask him what he meant about my taping our sessions.

He responds: "Oh, don't therapists usually record their sessions to play back later, or to share with other therapists?"

I ask him to say more and he tells me he imagines I play tapes of our sessions in front of a group of peers—men, he imagines—and they give me feedback about the work I do with him. I ask if he thinks I would tape our sessions without his consent.

Sean is silent for a minute or two, seems deep in thought, and grimaces. I ask what has come to mind and he tells me of an incident during high school when his girlfriend called him at home while several guys were visiting. He went into another room to pick up an extension and asked them to hang up. Instead, they listened to the conversation. For several days after that the guys who had been at his house mimicked Sean's "mushy" endearments whenever they passed him in the hall at school. He decided never to trust guys again. Telling me this story leads to a breakthrough in our relationship.

Sean is afraid of close contact with me, afraid that if he lets me really matter to him I will betray him, just like his friends did in high school. Of course, I would not have taped our conversations without getting Sean's consent. We examine Sean's reasons for assuming I might, and talk about ways he might, in the future, do a better job determining who he can trust and confide in.

Sean would like to leave his job and work part-time so he can spend more time with his daughter, but he is afraid other men might ridicule him for it. In other words, he is keeping up a tough front—the guy who is always battling to get ahead at work—just so that other guys will not laugh at him, presumably for being a loser. Of course, his tough front includes a certain amount of scorn he publicly exhibits for men who are not entirely manly.

Sean's fear of closeness with men leads to resistances in our therapeutic relationship, and therefore developments in our therapeutic relationship provide clues to Sean's inability to maintain close friendships. He complains about lacking "real" friends and wishes it were different:

"I think I'd like to have at least one really good friend, one whom I could trust entirely and have the kind of intense emotional interaction that I once had with my wife."

In other words, Sean secretly desires to have an intimacy with a man that reaches the level of trust and emotional intercourse that he has had only with his sexual partner. Once a therapist knows this, it is easy to decide what work lies ahead. Sean and I need to look at the kinds of things that hold him back in his search for friendships with men. Obviously the first hurdle for him is his fear that contemporary friends will reenact the high school scenario that was so unbearably painful.

I mentioned in Chapter Seven that the two patterns that regularly emerge in psychotherapies involving men—a battle for dominance and difficulty filling emotional space—also emerge in men's same-sex intimacies. I can help Sean transcend his distrust of a male therapist and learn about what intimacy and connection feel like. Perhaps he will seek out the same level of connection with other men. It is not so easy for men friends to have a discussion about the roots of their distrust and distancing. Of course, with no therapist present to make interpretations, one or both men would have to initiate a discussion of the way the relationship seems stuck. But friends do not give each other the same kind of sanction they give therapists to explore underlying motivations. Besides, men feel safer being vulnerable and taking risks with a therapist than they do with each other. Still, I believe that some of the same kinds of self-revelations that occur in the consulting room can occur in conversations between friends, but with friends neither member of the dyad speaks from a "neutral stance," and the exploration is mutual, not unidirectional.

To the friend I yelled at on the phone, I admitted that I never yelled at my brothers as a child, and consequently our sibling relationships lacked vitality. I told him I was glad this friendship, in contrast, was coming alive. He was then able to admit that my challenge made him feel he had been disloyal as a friend, and there were childhood precedents that made it very painful for him to hear that kind of criticism. We did not belabor the point. We had gotten past a barrier to deeper intimacy, and did not want to overly psychologize our relationship. But the mutual personal sharing helped us understand each other and reach the kind of understanding that we needed in order to get past the angry outburst.

Men's Foibles, Women's Example

There are as many stories as there are men. One man tells me he had good buddies in high school and college and does not know why he just has not been in touch with them or made new friends in so many years; another tells me he never was able to sustain friendships. One man says he was never able to relate to his father and that is why he cannot relate to other men; another tells me he was very close to his father but still has no close friends. Other men—the lucky few—have very close friends. David Michaelis (1983) interviewed men who had "exceptional friendships," and found that even these men's frienships were limited; for instance, they tended to avoid talk of competition and sex. In general, men admit that friendship is problematic.

Drury Sherrod (1987) reviews the literature and reports on his interviews with several hundred male and female college students about their friendships, concluding that:

> For most men, most of the time, the dimension of intimacy in friendships with other men may be irrelevant to their lives. According to the research, men seek not intimacy but companionship, not disclosure but commitment. Men's friendships involve unquestioned acceptance rather than unrestricted affirmation. When men are close, they achieve closeness through shared

activities, and on the basis of shared activities, men infer intimacy simply because they are friends. Yet, there are times when a man becomes aware that something is lacking. (pp. 221–223)

McGill (1985) found that most of the 700 men she interviewed lack close friends. Daniel Levinson (1978) found close friendship to be rare among the men he interviewed for his classic study on the stages of adult life. Sherrod believes men once enjoyed very close friendships— in classical Greece or post-Renaissance Europe, for instance—and then, because of historical changes in worklife, marriage, and urban culture, men grew distant from each other in terms of personal relations. Hammond and Jablow (1987) suggest that close male friendships have always been more of a myth than a reality.

There is this familiar scenario: a heterosexual man retreats into his couple relationship, gets his emotional needs met there, and feels satisfied. The woman, meanwhile, seeks out close friends outside the marriage. This scenario develops, in most cases, because the woman has a greater need to maintain close same-sex friendships even when she is in a primary relationship whereas the man finds it harder—for all the reasons I have mentioned—to make and keep friends, and is more willing to focus his emotional energy on a single partner. Lillian Rubin (1983, 1985) interviewed married couples about their friendships and discovered that the women had many more and deeper same-sex friendships; over two-thirds of the men could not name a best friend other than their wives whereas a large majority of the women could easily name a best friend of the same sex. There are many exceptions, of course. For instance there are women who cut off their friends when they get involved with a man and there are men who maintain very close lifetime friendships and see their men friends even after they get married. But in the more typical situation where the man cuts off his friends while the woman retains close same-sex friendships, the discrepancy eventually leads to problems in the primary relationship. Perhaps the man feels threatened by the woman's independent relationships and activities. Or, when they fight she has her friends to go to for support while he feels he has no one to talk to.

This is the point at which men resort to psychotherapy—but, as I mentioned at the end of Chapter Seven, instead of helping the man patch things up with his partner and returning him to the same situation, it might be useful for the therapist to examine how and why he has become so isolated and dependent exclusively on his female partner, and help him develop a richer network of intimates. Straight men's tendency to talk about their emotional life exclusively with women means there is little vitality when they are with each other, and explains why the male culture of work and public life is relatively cold and lonely. But men are just plain difficult to be intimate with—if one is a man, that is.

Robert Bly and Michael Meade (Bly, 1989) claim that "the male mode of feeling" is very different than the female mode; for instance, men are not as interested in face-to-face discussions of personal matters, preferring instead to stand shoulder-to-shoulder facing a common task or adversary. The point is valid, men do have different ways. When women writers mock male shoulder-to-shoulder relating and imply that face-to-face relationships are the only kind that are truly intimate, they alienate men who might otherwise listen to what women are trying to tell them about the value of sharing personal stories. At the same time, shoulder-to-shoulder intimacies can be rather limiting, and men would do well to learn more about the face-to-face variety. The story-telling that occurs at men's gatherings is a move in the right direction. Men also have much to learn from women about friendship—as long as they keep in mind that men's friendships are different, of course.

Carol Gilligan (1982) contrasts the man's quest for status in a hierarchy with the woman's for connection with others. She believes women seek to be the center of a web of relationships:

> Thus the images of hierarchy and web inform different modes of assertion and response: the wish to be alone at the top and the consequent fear that others will get too close; the wish to be at the center of connection and the consequent fear of being too far out on the edge. (p. 63)

Men who seek closer intimacies are quite regularly forced to reevaluate their priorities. Close friendships require a certain amount of time spent together, and sometimes there is not enough time in the day to work long hours, be with one's family, and keep in touch with friends.

Lillian Rubin (1985) explores the differences between men's and women's friendships and writes:

> Generally, women's friendships with each other rest on shared intimacies, self-revelation, nurturance and emotional support. In contrast, men's relationships are marked by shared activities. (p. 61)

She proceeds to describe a man who is exceptional in that he has a very close male friend. But when his wife has an affair, he does not tell his friend. "Why not?," Lillian asks. The man responds:

It's just not something I could talk about, that's all. Hell, I don't know. I was hurt and ashamed and angry, and I felt like crying and like killing her and the son-of-a-bitch who got her involved, who was a guy I knew. How could I tell anybody all that?. (pp. 67–68)

In explaining the differences between men's and women's friendships, Rubin mentions the obvious—that girls are rewarded for expressing their feelings and enjoying nurturing relationships while boys are taught to hide any sign of weakness and neediness. She emphasizes the singularly formative role of the child's early relationship with the mother and, in the boy's case, the consequences of having to "dis-identify" with her so abruptly during the Oedipal stage of development (see Chapter Three). A problem with Rubin's formulation is her assumption that gendered identity formation occurs very early, and mainly in the context of the mother–infant dyad. The role of the father and of later events is minimized. Compare this with Peter Blos' (1984, see Chapter Six) formulation about fathers and sons wherein he emphasizes the "negative Oedipal triangle," the very young son's love for the nurturing father, and his wish to be just like him. Blos insists that the events of adolescence can be as formative of one's gender identity as can one's early childhood, and I heartily concur.

Stuart Miller (1983) reports that many men are secretly envious of women's ability to truly enjoy their friends. He writes:

A wife, touched by the women's movement perhaps, begins to form serious engagements with other women. You hear her talking on the phone as you watch television at night. Politely, she gets up and closes the door so you won't be disturbed. But you are, somehow, even more disturbed. Occasionally you hear the sound of a peculiarly hearty laughter that you don't have in your own life, laughter of a kind that your wife doesn't even share with you. A shadow falls across your consciousness but you don't know exactly what to do about it. You respect her new friendships but you are envious. (p.32)

I have learned quite a lot about friendship from women. For instance, I have learned how two friends can be very angry at each other, call each other names, and then when calm returns go on being close friends. More typical of male friendships is one-fight-and-it's-over. I felt terrible after that first fight I described with my friend, I was certain there was something wrong with me, a certain meanness. I felt this even though, when my wife has the same kind of argument with a woman friend, I support her and tell her I admire the way she can be so forthright, fierce, and forgiving, and deepen her intimacies in the process. But somehow, for me, the rules are different. A man is not supposed to be so emotional and demanding.

The Unwritten Rules of Male Friendship

There are unwritten rules that guide men's approach to same-sex friendships. High on the list is the one about reciprocity (Pasick, 1990). For instance, one man invites another to lunch, they have a good time and the first man awaits a reciprocal invitation from the second. It does not come. The first man is stuck. Should he wait for the other's invitation to meet again, or break protocol and call him a second time? Men too often adhere to a tit-for-tat rule and cut off the relationship. I have recently changed my mind about how to proceed when I get into this situation. Instead of letting my feeling of rejection take over and swearing never to make any further effort to befriend a man who has failed to reciprocate my first invitation to lunch, I am now willing to call men I would like to get to know two or three times without receiving a return call. Then, in subtle or not so subtle terms, I let the other man know that it hurts my feelings that he does not call to initiate contact and that I will not keep doing all the initiating forever. Either he needs to take some initiative in this friendship or I will give up the struggle. Men who hear me, who are willing to engage with me about such things, are the most likely to make good friends.

If men cannot break free of the tit-for-tat sensibility, we will repeatedly get stuck at the beginning of intimacies and never get really close. We will never get to the conversation where one man confronts the other:

"I'm a little hurt—last time we got together I told you my mother was about to undergo major surgery and you never called to see how she is doing. And, by the way, how come I had to call you to make this lunch date—I called to initiate our last lunch, why don't you reciprocate?"

If such things are said in the right tone, at a time when the other man is able to hear the caring side of the message, perhaps he can accept the criticism and admit that he, like most men, is not very adept at keeping in touch with other men. In general, whenever we are able to find an unstated rule that inhibits men's intimacies, it helps to identify it and consciously circumvent or renegotiate that rule—consciously pushing past the reciprocity rule is one example.

A second unwritten rule involves trust. It is as if men were saying to each other, "if you cross me once it's all over." This rule originates in the Wyatt Earp, back-to-the-door mentality that is so much a part of male culture. As I mentioned in Chapter Seven, men feel they need to size each other up if they are to avoid "being shafted." This is one of the ways our competitive, dog-eat-dog social relations constrict our possibilities for deep intimacy. And as soon as there is a sign of danger, the man is out of the relationship. Men do not make up. It is easier to drop a friend—or decide never to trust him again—than it is to stand toe-to-toe with a man and holler about the way he has hurt one's feelings or betrayed one. And then there is always the threat of violence. Above all else, men do not back down—another unwritten rule—so why should either man expect to get anywhere in a confrontation? It is easier to look for another friend.

The third rule: one does not cross the line of male propriety. Robert Pasick (1990) includes in his list of issues that prevent men from maintaining close same-sex relationships homophobia and men's adherence to a narrow definition of "masculinity." Men are stiff with each other. Of course there are pats on the butt after a football victory—if those huge professional linemen can slap each others' buttocks exuberantly, why cannot any male sports enthusiast smack any other enthusiast's backside? So we set up a more complicated, but still unstated rule: "real men" do not exhibit excessive affection toward each other in public, with the exception that an exuberant hug or slap on the buttocks is okay at victory time.

A fourth rule: A man does not expose his raw emotional experience if there is a chance there will be no response. As a male client tells me: "You don't want to get caught with your ass dangling out there." Stuart Miller (1983) describes his experience attempting to get a friend, Ronald, to talk about his feelings:

> He is a happy, self-contained character, a man who knows himself and is at peace. But what am I? A strange kind of needy creature, with hankerings after some sort of closeness that others don't seem to require? Wanting to be known, to share something, a brother, trust—I'm not even sure I know what it is that I want, much less how to get it. And what will the other man think? He will, he does, slight me after I put myself forward. My pride is put into question by this needing and reaching. I know these feelings and I must fight them all the while that I do this crazy thing. It is heroic, in a small way, what I am doing. I know that, too. (p. 45)

Most men lack Miller's perseverance and give up on developing close male friendships.

Again, the lessons from therapy can be applied to men's same-sex intimacies. While discussing men's difficulties filling emotional space (Chapter Seven) I shared my therapeutic strategy: I look for moments of real aliveness in the therapeutic encounter and then ask why there are not more moments like that. In sharp contrast, men tend to steer clear of tensions and animosities in their friendships, and deaden their interactions in the process. For instance a client, Keith, tells me about a friend who continually talks about himself every time they meet and asks Keith no questions about himself. I ask why Keith continues to get together with this friend and he tells me that it is a lot of fun to be with him, and they have been friends for a long time. We try to figure out how Keith might confront his friend about what he perceives as self-centeredness. Keith asks his friend to lunch and confronts him about the fact that he never asks Keith any questions. The friend listens, and then asks why it should be his responsibility to do so, why cannot Keith volunteer something about himself? Keith thinks for a minute and then agrees, he does too much waiting to be asked and could volunteer more. Then the friend also agrees that he is too self-centered. He says he is glad Keith had the courage to confront him. In the ensuing months, the two get together on several occasions and Keith reports to me that their interactions are more lively and mutually rewarding than ever.

Even men who have joined men's groups, attend men's gatherings, and consider themselves part of the men's movement continue to have conflicts about friendship. How many men are in men's groups, meeting every other week or monthly with a bunch of guys, but never seeing other members outside of group meetings? The same question could be asked about men's gatherings. The logical conclusion is that men do not go to each other in times of need, only on scheduled occasions, and this means there can be very limited spontaneity and dependency in the encounter.

Gay men, on the average, experience more vitality in their same-sex relationships than do straight men. Is this because there is the possibility of sex? Is it because they have gotten used to the stigma that goes along with public displays of affection between men and consequently can permit themselves to be more spontaneous and demonstrative than straight men who live in dread of that kind of stigma? There are many possible explanations. Whatever the reason, gay men tell me they do not experience the deadness in their same-sex friendships that straight men experience in theirs. I am mentioning a trend, not a hard-and-fast rule. There are many exceptions, of course. Gay men are teaching straight men a lot about being intimate with men. There is the danger gay men will resent being always the instructor—straight men have to develop more expertise in the art of male friendship, too—but for now, the leadership of gay men in this pursuit serves as another good reason for an alliance between gays and straights in the struggle to change gender relations.

Rewriting the Rules for Male Friendship

A male friend is having problems in his marriage. We talk. I am a very active listener, asking many questions. A day later I call to see how he is. A few days later I call again. He is not very forthcoming about his situation when we talk on the phone, and never initiates any phone conversations or further meetings. I wonder if I am being too intrusive. I decide to wait for him to contact me. Many months pass. Then he calls me and we meet for lunch. He tells me he has been going through big changes, and things are much better. His marriage is the best it has ever been. He has decided to enter psychotherapy to explore some of the underlying issues. I say good, and by the way, I was angry about the way he broke off contact. (I know, why didn't I say that then?—but it was a situation where I called him three or four times, he never returned my calls, I figured I was being too intrusive, and backed off.) He explains that he was working things out on his own, something I know about all too well, and had been planning to reestablish contact.

Then he tells me that something I said in our initial conversation put him off. Hesitantly, he proceeds to tell me, fearing my feelings will be hurt, that when we spoke and he was on the verge of a break-up I told him about a mutual friend who had had an affair. He feared that, if he told me what was going on with him, I would betray his confidence and tell someone else about his personal crisis. Here was a very complicated issue. As a therapist, I am well versed in keeping confidences. As a matter of fact, I had thought about the issue and decided this mutual friend would not have minded—perhaps I was wrong. But there is another issue. I challenged him with the logic of his criticism: if, when a primary relationship is in trouble, we do not want anyone to know, and for that reason cut off all our friends (as Rubin's interviewee had done when his wife was having an affair), and then we go to see a couple therapist with the partner, does not that close off an important dimension of friendship and limit the depth of intimacy? Men have a tendency to make personal crises an all too private matter. Then we go to see therapists trusting that they will maintain confidentiality.

Parenthetically, this negotiation between friends illustrates the "dual potential of psychotherapy" (Kupers, 1986), the utility as well as the limitations of therapy. We visit therapists, on the average, because we find our community and our network of intimates lacking in important ways. And therapy helps us refashion our coping skills and improve our intimacies as well as our sense of self. But the more we place our trust in professionals and their pledge of confidentiality, the less pressure there is for us to struggle with our friends and other intimates to establish a deeper basis for trust. Thus, psychotherapy can help us develop the capacity for close friendship (Gordon & Pasick, 1990), or it can serve to subvert our need for friends. For many men, the therapist becomes the trusted one and there is consequently less need to challenge friends when they are untrustworthy. This issue warrants further discussion, in intimate dyads as well as in men's groups and gatherings.

Perhaps we can collectively rewrite the rules so that we will be able to talk to each other about personal matters, balancing the need to protect confidentiality with the need to avoid isolation. Each time my wife and I have a serious dispute, I know a number of her friends will know the bloody details, and sometimes I feel self-conscious in their presence because of it. But, at the same time, I am glad she has the support of good friends. Men are more likely to suffer alone, afraid to tell others the unpleasant details of their relational upheavals for fear that the secrets that are disclosed at a time of crisis might be used against them.

In this case, my issue with my friend was that I was afraid he had avoided me in his moment of need because I was too intrusive, so I planned to wait until he contacted me again. But then resentment grew when he did not seek me out. For his part, he did not feel strong enough to voice his concern about confidentiality and my trustworthiness, and to confront me about it so he could decide whether I was someone he might safely confide in. It turns out he also wondered if I would keep secrets from my wife about him. At the end of our conversation about all this he agreed men are all too private, gave me permission to tell my wife about our conversation, and it was left to me to say I would not tell my wife all he had told me, but would exercise the kind of discretion I felt he would want.

Having had this confrontation in one relationship, I felt obligated to return to the man whose affair I had mentioned to see if he objected to my breaching whatever unspoken vow of confidentiality had been implicit in our earlier discussions. I discovered that we did not share the same notion of confidentiality. Perhaps because I am a therapist, I assumed that when a man tells another about something as personal as an affair, there is an implicit vow of confidentiality. Does that vow preclude my sharing the fact of the affair with my wife, who this man knows very well? This, too, is uncharted terrain and requires some negotiation. When I told this friend that I had told another man, a mutual friend, about the affair, he was neither surprised nor upset. I had shared his confidence because the other friend was in the midst of a terrible marital storm and, though he was not having an affair, it looked bad for the marriage. I wanted to let him know that another man—the friend who had the affair—had come back from even worse marital discord and reestablished a very deep romantic connection with his partner. In other words, I wanted to inject some hope into this friend's thinking about his marriage. The friend who had the affair understood my motive and told me he was glad I was able to use his affair as an example of how far out of phase relationships can go and still return to a deep connectedness. Here we are, three male friends, working out the ground rules for our intimacies.

Each man has to overcome a different hurdle vis à vis friendship. What unifies us is the fact that there always are those hurdles. We share a certain amount of collective incapability in the realm of man-to-man relating. Each of us has our own foibles that contribute to the collective incapability. And I am optimistic about the future, largely because so many men are embarking on a course of "men's work" to help them be more open and trusting. But if we are to transcend our collective incapability, then we must discuss the whole issue and, essentially, rewrite the unstated social rules for being friends.

CHAPTER NINE

The Men's Movement:
Making the Personal Political

The men's movement is divided. Some men believe that merely by meeting together—in psychotherapy, in men's groups, or in men's gatherings and conferences—they can discover the secret of "being a man" and dramatically improve their situation. This group includes psychologists who do "men's work," men who lead and participate in large workshops and subscribe to the "mythopoetic" school of thought, "men's rights" advocates including divorce reformers, a large number of men who are in recovery from drug, alcohol, and other addictions, and men who have survived childhood incest and abuse. Another group, the "political" or "pro-feminist" segment of the men's movement, believes it is the inequities inherent in our social relations that cause men's difficulties, that one cannot change one gender's plight without changing the relations between genders, and that straight men just join with women and gays in a struggle to radically transform those restrictive social relations.

The split is reminiscent of the 1960s when one large group of activists believed the righteous struggle was a political one to end racism, war, and poverty while another large group could not tolerate the personal relationships that evolved among the activists and instead created a youth-oriented counterculture. There were attempts to mend the split between those who wanted to concentrate on political struggles and those who wanted to evolve new forms of personal life, including the notion that the personal is political.

The women's movement has survived from that era and thrived, in large part because women have succeeded to a significant extent in making the personal political. Of course, women share a common oppression, which serves to unite them. There is less unity among men. This is not only because "men are the oppressors," though that is an issue men must eventually confront. It is more a matter of men's proclivity to compete for dominance. Men have trouble agreeing on anything because each would like to convince the others he has the sole correct answer to what ails us. So we argue.

The current divisions of the men's movement bring to mind another movement's rift, the splits that erupted in 1912 between Sigmund Freud and his two brilliant collaborators, Carl Jung and Alfred Adler (Gay, 1988). It was an unfortunate parting of ways. Freud was the brilliant scientist, philosopher, and clinical strategist. Jung was more in touch with the creative spirit, the meaning of myths, and the mystery and magic of the unconscious. Adler explored the social roots of each individual's feelings of inadequacy, and the "masculine protest" that serves to compensate men for their deeply felt sense of inferiority. If these three pioneers of psychoanalysis were alive today, I imagine Freud might be a leader among therapists who do "men's work," Jung would certainly be among the mythopoets, and Adler would likely feel at home among the "political" or "pro-feminist" sector of the men's movement. Perhaps, if the three had continued to collaborate in spite of theoretical differences and personality clashes, we would have a more unified theory of psyche, soul and society than we have today.

Psychotherapists explain men's feelings of emptiness and inadequacy in relation to early childhood deprivation, the mythopoetic section of the men's movement argues that the psychologists and the "political" men lack soul and vitality; and the "political men" claim that therapists and mythopoets are ethnocentric and lack politics. Let us assume that there is a kernel of truth in all three claims, and that we must combine all three approaches if we are to have an effective men's movement. In other words, the men's movement must relate to the personal needs that cause men to seek change (including the personal sense of inadequacy that makes men feel threatened by powerful women, the need to find meaning in one's life, and the need to express one's spirituality), while remaining aware of the social tragedies that are unfolding in front of our eyes (including the widening gap between rich and poor, high unemployment, unbridled racism, homophobia and sexism, homelessness, the destruction of the environment, and the constant threat of war). In this chapter I will examine the strengths and shortcomings of the psychological/psychotherapeutic, the mythopoetic/spiritual, and the political/pro-feminist approaches, and suggest that an integration of all three is needed if we are to redefine power and significantly restructure gender roles and gender relations.

The Psychological Approach and the
Dual Potential of Psychotherapy

Herbert Marcuse (1955) theorized the dual potential of psychoanalysis and psychotherapy in his discussion of repressive desublimation. In order to demonstrate the elusiveness of the notion of social progress, he played on two psychoanalytic terms: repression and sublimation. Sublimation is the diversion of psychic (instinctual) energy from sexual to nonsexual aims, for instance, from erotic fantasies into creative ventures. Freud believed that repression of sexual impulses was at the core of the neuroses, and he viewed sublimation as a way to channel the impulses into socially accepted activities. Of course, in Freud's Vienna, massive repression of sexuality was socially sanctioned, in fact prescribed. Many early analysts, particularly Wilhelm Reich (1945), believed that a lessening of culturally mandated sexual repression would free people from neurotic constrictions and at the same time bring about social progress.

Since Freud's day, sexuality has become part of public life. Sex is explored openly in the cinema, manipulated by advertising, taught to the young, and discussed in newspapers and magazines. Are the younger generations who are immersed in explicit sexuality from a very tender age any more free of neurotic constrictions, or any more ready to make a revolution, than were those who learned to repress sexuality in Freud's day? There may no longer be the same need to sublimate; the forms of neurosis and character structure may change; but sex thus "de-sublimated" can still be "repressive"—this to the extent consumers are programmed to desire and fantasize about *Playboy* bunnies and movie stars, for instance, in the service of commodity sales. Marcuse's point is that there is no single event or advance that represents progress in any absolute sense. What is progress at one moment or in one context may well become the new form of repression in the next. In fact, built into contemporary social relations is a tendency to co-opt seemingly subversive developments and weave them into the fabric of existing commodity relations.

I have presented an example of the dual potential of psychotherapy in regard to friendship (Chapter Eight). Therapy can help men transcend their personal blocks and be better friends; at the same time reliance on a therapist diminishes the urgency of a man's need to take time out from a busy schedule and develop same-sex intimacies. Elsewhere I discuss therapy's dual potential in relation to the widespread practice of brief psychotherapy (Kupers, 1986).

"Men's work" is the latest rubric of the therapy world. Everyone seems to be doing it, women therapists as well as men. A plethora of books have been published on male psychology, men's dreams, men in therapy, and so forth. There are leaderless men's groups, and there are those that are run by therapists. Ideally, on the positive side of therapy's dual potential, therapy can help men reclaim their vitality and power in interpersonal relationships without becoming sexist. Therapy can also help men be more in touch with their feelings, more open with others, and more spontaneous. It can help men work through unresolved conflicts with their fathers, as well as their ambivalence about being a father. Men in therapy can process their conflicts about work and ambition and seek a work place that makes them feel comfortable. And therapy can help men transcend their obsession with pornography and their conflicts about homosexuality. All of these functions of therapy weigh in heavily on the progressive side of therapy's dual potential.

On the other side, immersion in psychotherapy tends to direct one's gaze inward, away from social problems. James Hillman (1990), a Jungian analyst who has become a leader of the mythopoetic men's movement, says it very well:

> Why are the intelligent people—at least among the white middle class—so passive now? Because the sensitive, intelligent people are in therapy! They've been in therapy in the United States for 30, 40 years, and during that time there's been a tremendous political decline in this country.

Psychotherapy turns our gaze inward as we search for the childhood precedents of our current tragedies or the deeper meaning of our problems being intimate. Meanwhile, social problems are ignored by a numbed populace.

Another Jungian who is popular at men's gatherings is Robert Moore (Moore & Gillette, 1990). His approach is the opposite of Hillman's:

> Ours is a psychological age rather than an institutional one. What used to be done for us by institutional structures and through ritual process, we now have to do inside ourselves, for ourselves. Ours is a culture of the individual rather than the collective. (p. 45)

Moore grasps the problem correctly—it is our extreme individualism. But unlike Hillman he leaves the social problem untouched as he instructs the privileged few how to cope with our hyper-individualistic status quo.

The clinician is constantly making a choice: focus entirely inward or integrate the inner dynamics with due consideration of contemporary social reality. I hear a certain list of complaints from a client in therapy. I can check the list against the known symptoms of a mental disorder—for instance depression or narcissistic personality—and begin to analyze the childhood roots of a man's narcissism; or I can think about the man's complaints in the context of social events. Some clinicians have attempted to integrate psychological and social concerns in their theories and clinical practices, including Alfred Adler (1927), Wilhelm Reich (1972), Erich Fromm (1962), Franz Fanon (1965), Franco Basaglia (1980), R. D. Laing (1967), The Radical Therapist Collective (1971), Jean Baker Miller (1976), and Joel Kovel (1981). It is relatively easy to demonstrate the interconnections of psychological and social themes in the lives of actual men, if the therapist chooses to do so. Gender issues, in particular, touch on the interconnections.

Roger walks into my office for the first time just after hitting his wife. He insists: "It was only a slap with an open hand, she's making too much of it."

He is convinced that if he does not seek therapy she will leave him forever. Of course, if she had not insisted, he would never have come to see a psychiatrist. A part of him believes her current ultimatum is just another of her "histrionic stances," and will "blow over," just like the half dozen other times he has hit her during their five years together.

"Then why did you come to see me—couldn't you just wait out the storm?" I ask.

"Yeah, but something's different this time. I think she might really leave me."

Honesty—a beginning—perhaps a toehold. If I can only maintain some semblance of neutrality, perhaps I can reach this man. But I am repelled by his sexism, the way he can brutalize a woman and worry only about whether she will leave him. At this point, I am not even certain I can work with him.

Weeks pass. He and his wife make up. He begins to like therapy. He tells me he is frightened of losing control again. We explore the roots of his uncontrollable rage, tracing it back to his relationship with an alcoholic mother. He was angry at her for never driving him to school and for never visiting his school and meeting his teachers. Maybe he was even angry at her for deserting him, leaving him at school when he was so ill-prepared to be there. When he entered kindergarten he did not know how to relate to other kids—he had spent his whole life alone at home with his mother, and there he was left to his own devices while she turned to the bottle. He was rejected by the other kids, and beaten by bullies. He did not know how to play the games. Meanwhile he longed to be home with his mother.

Roger attempted to cope, acting the loner at school, shying away from games and activities. But after the first few beatings, whenever someone tried to bully him, he lost his temper. He fought often, and beat up many opponents. He never was in any real trouble—a few suspensions, a warning here and there. By the time he entered high school he had learned to be more sociable, almost popular, and had his temper under control. In his early twenties, he lived with a woman for a year. He loved her. She left him. He beat her up. This outburst of violence frightened him, but he quickly forgot about it. His present relationship began just after that.

I ask if there is a temporal sequence to his loss of control.

"I've never thought about it in those terms. Let me think."

He ponders a moment. Then he remembers that the day he hit his wife was the day he had been unfairly penalized at work because he had failed to get an assignment done on time. He begins to make connections. He left work in a rage, came home, and started a fight with his wife.

"As if it was her fault," he adds solemnly.

This realization leads to the next: he always blamed his mother for the beatings he received on the school yard. At this point Roger recalls another relevant childhood memory: his father drank and argued loudly with his mother, occasionally beating her. This occurred in front of the boy, who was overwhelmed by a mixture of rage, fear, and impotence.

Where is the questioning to be turned at this point? Should we explore the early dynamics further? The mixture of rage, fear, and impotence he felt watching his father beat his mother? Or should we turn attention to the social context, the unfairness of the hierarchy at work, the economic realities of speedups and layoffs? Too often therapy proceeds as if by formula: first, the personal history and important intimacies are examined, then psychodynamic formulations are established, and finally the client's perceptions of the larger picture are analyzed in terms of the psychodynamics. For instance a therapist might point out that while Roger's complaints about unfairness at work may be well founded, the thing to note is that his relationship with his supervisor resembles that with his father. This selective attention occurs in the name of therapeutic neutrality.

Of course, there are important events in Roger's past. His father, a factory worker like Roger, drank and beat Roger's mother after being fired or docked pay at work. He displaced his impotent rage from the workplace to the home, and like Roger, he was unaware of doing so. In other words, he provided the model for Roger's displacement. By encouraging Roger to focus on his early internalization of an abusive father, a therapist would be directing Roger to find the roots of his uncontrollable rage entirely inside his own psyche. Michael Lerner (1991) points out the role of the American dream in all of this. If we believe that each individual has the potential to strike it rich and become an Andrew Carnegie or John Rockefeller, then each individual's failure to do so is attributable solely to his personal deficiencies. It was the depth to which the American dream was inscribed within the American psyche that made it so easy for psychotherapy to become an indispensable way of life for so many Americans.

It is a fact that, because of identifiable trends in the economy, plants like Roger's are speeding up their production lines or closing. The threat of the latter is used to attain worker compliance in the former. The management of Roger's plant is resorting to authoritarian methods to enforce the speedup, methods that tend to evoke feelings of impotence and humiliation among workers. I opt to discuss this with Roger, and then extrapolate back in time and talk about how Roger's father's brutality was likewise reactive to an alienating work experience. Roger is ready to grasp the crucial difference: whereas his father felt impotent and could do nothing about it except drink and beat his mother, and whereas Roger actually was impotent as a child in terms of protecting his mother, he is now an adult and in a much better position to do something constructive about this kind of harassment at work. By admitting how bad he feels about being abusive at home, Roger is able to uncover a psychosocial dynamic that explains his misdirected rage. He decides to play a more active role in his union's struggle to end the speedup, thus hoping to diminish the humiliation he feels. And he is able to talk about all this with his wife and arrive at a new level of resolve not to abuse her in the future.

Roger's dilemma is not unique. Wife-beating, child abuse, and incest are widespread. Too often therapists focus on the psychopathology and childhood antecedents in explaining domestic violence and abuse, failing to recognize social variables such as unemployment and the kind of underemployment and demeaning work that deprive a man of his self-respect. Such conditions do not excuse the perpetrator and they do not entirely explain his motivation to abuse, but they are important considerations nonetheless, and can be a productive topic for exploration, in therapy and in the men's movement. Working with men who abuse women and children is hard work, and I deeply respect the clinicians and counselors who are dedicated to providing this sorely needed service. For a review of their work, see Warters (1991). Of course, in doing this work, men must be accountable to the victims and the women who run shelters for battered women; at all costs we must minimize the liklihood that the batterer will be put through a counseling program only to return to his partner, supposedly "changed," and proceed to batter her again. The National Organization for Men Against Sexism (NOMAS) task force on Ending Men's Violence is developing a framework for collaboration between men and women doing this kind of work.

Men are taxed heavily by the burdens of success and power. Is it any wonder there are disturbingly high rates of suicide, heart attack, hypertension, incarceration, loneliness, and depression in men? Men who can afford the fees consult therapists for advice about all of this. Thus there is a dual potential in psychotherapy and "men's work": it can serve to prop up the American dream and the idea that those of us who do not strike it rich are suffering from an inner flaw, or it can serve to give us the strength to break free of this defeatist attitude.

Men's Gatherings and Mythopoets

Men's gatherings are not new. Lionel Tiger (1969) chronicles the evolution of men's groups and gatherings from prehistoric times to the present. Today men gather in union halls, athletic fields, on picket lines, in boardrooms, at conventions, in demonstrations against racism and war, and so forth. What is new is for men to gather for the express purpose of figuring out what it means to be a man. Why don't we know that? Why do men experience a need to gather in the woods, to drum and to create rituals? It seems obvious that men are trying in these ways to fill a void in their lives. The men who gather say that in their routine lives men lack fellowship, spirituality, a meaning larger than themselves and their everyday pursuits, and a sense of their own vitality and worthiness (Erkel, 1990; Shewey, 1992; Stanton, 1991). They turn to the leaders of the men's movement for wisdom and they gather together to begin to experience mentorship, initiation, and a new kind of brotherhood. It feels good to be at such gatherings. It is fun to dance with men, to hug, to tell one's story. It even breaks down some of the posturing and intellectuality.

Shepherd Bliss borrowed the term "mythopoetic" from philosophy (where it refers to the pre-Hellenic oral tradition) and applied it to contemporary men's pursuits. Bliss (1990) says it is:

the remythologizing of masculinity. The looking back to the old stories for our contemporary times. New images, new metaphors— and old ones. Because there's a lot of confusion about what it means to be a man.

Bliss goes on to say:

> When somebody dies, you cry and you grieve. But in our society we put these spells on men. We tell them big boys don't cry. Don't lean on me. Stiff upper lip. And what we need to do is break these spells. We need to remember what those exact words put on you as a man to repress you were. What were the gestures that your parents, school-teachers made and how can you free yourself of them? That's why we use storytelling, poetry, drumming, dance— to break those kinds of spells. (pp. xx)

Men "in recovery" flock to men's gatherings. They suffer from the same gender traps that afflict nonaddicts, and they are aware that they fled into addiction while trying desparately to fill the void they felt in the center of their souls. Phil Z (1990) discusses the warm collaboration between C. G. Jung and Bill W, the founder of Alcoholics Anonymous (Alcoholics Anonymous, 1939) and explains:

> The alcoholic drinks, despite the indisputable evidence that he should not, to ameliorate the psychological and spiritual suffering resulting from the loss of contact between his ego and Higher Self. The obsession to drink grows out of a misguided effort to satisfy what is, in essence, a spiritual thirst. (p. 210)

Men's gatherings offer a spiritual community, a "ritual space," and a safe place to vent all the feelings that had been trapped for so many years inside a traditional male persona or drowned in a bottle.

Terrence O'Connor (1990) reports on a large, week-long gathering he attended:

> And there is sharing. Sometime during the week nearly every man stands and bares his heart to the group. The pain is breaking through. The burdens of isolation are dropped. Most of the sharing is about fathers and grandfathers, but some is of a more immediate nature. One construction worker, a man in his fifties, stands up and tells us that in all his life he had never let another man get physically close to him. This morning in mask-making his partner had touched his face with gentle fingers, and, here he chokes up, "and I like it." He bursts into tears. He is immediately surrounded by comforting men. (p. 38)

Of course men who so desire have every right to play drums, dance together and get in touch with those inner kings, warriors and wildmen, and there is much to be gained by creating new ways for men to be together. The question is, should we stop there? Will we continue to leave those weekend gatherings and return home to an unchanged world? Will we continue to lose touch with each other between meetings, as men traditionally do, or will we establish new ways for men to be intimate on a day-to-day basis? What of political issues and social movements? What about sexism? How can men play a role in changing what ails us as a gender and as a society?

Unless men who are trying to create new forms of masculinity pay serious attention to the power relationships that shape the experience of both genders, men's meetings with each other will result in little more than nontraditional forms for male encounters. When I hear leaders in the men's movement say that the problem is that women have become too powerful and men have lost the power they once had, I begin to worry about the possiblity that the men's movement might take a bad turn, a turn toward backlash and the reassertion of male dominance in a new guise. Susan Faludi (1991) is worried about this possibility, too. She demonstrates convincingly that, contrary to claims that women have won their freedom in the last twenty years and that it is their victory that causes problems such as partnerlessness and the feminization of poverty, women are actually far from winning the battle for equal rights and it is the same old garden variety sexism that holds women back today.

The reason men have lost their way is not that women are beginning to find theirs. Women's success in claiming a voice and a place for themselves in the public arena should be cause for men to celebrate, not a reason for men to shudder and blame women for men's feelings of inadequacy. Tony Astrachan (1986) reports on his interviews with men of all classes and races who feel their lives have been improved on account of women's gains. A large number of men realize that their feelings of inadequacy stem from the state of the economy, the requirement that men fight for dominance in a ruthless rat race if they are to feel like "real men," and the lack of any real say in this society's political direction.

The men's movement is also subject to the laws of repressive desublimation. I have mentioned the progressive potential, for instance the opportunity to collaborate closely with other men in the creation of a new kind of community. Sharing our stories offers us an opportunity to rewrite them together. The energy that is generated at men's gatherings is a welcome alternative to men's isolation and inability to fill emotional space with each other. And the mythopoetic men's movement is becoming fiercely protective of the environment and the Earth, and opposed to wars of aggression.

But there is a dual potential in the creation of new rituals. On the one hand, there is the attempt to reclaim ageless wisdom about the conduct of lives that was passed on in myths and rituals until recent generations when change became the byword and tradition receded from our cultural life. Many people believe that by rediscovering the myths of the past we can salvage that ageless wisdom and find a more grounded path for ourselves in today's tumultuous world. On the other hand, especially when the traditions come from a past of patriarchal domination and the myths were collected from the only class that had access to the written word—Greek patricians, the aristocrats of Old England and Europe, and so forth—the values of the past, including racism, sexism, and homophobia, are passed along with the wisdom.

An example of patriarchal bias is this description of the warrior archetype by Robert Moore and Douglas Gillette (1990):

> The Warrior energy, then, no matter what else it may be, is indeed universally present in us men and in the civilizations we create, defend, and extend. It is a vital ingredient in our world-building and plays an important role in extending the benefits of the highest human virtues and cultural achievements to all of humanity. (p. 79)

I see nothing wrong with giving the warrior energy its due. But I do not believe that men are biologically fated to make war. Erich Fromm (1973) and Ashley Montagu (1968) debunked this biologistic bias many years ago, and it is alarming to find it reappearing in the new men's literature. Moore and Gillette rationalize wars of empire on the basis of spreading "higher" human virtues, as if the peoples and nations that have been plundered and raped by successive waves of advancing warrior nations throughout history did not have valuable cultures of their own. Have the lives of Native Americans improved since their conquest by European-American warriors?

A striking characteristic of late capitalism is the tendency for people to be alienated from various aspects of what we consider most human, and then for those aspects of humanness to reappear as commodities one can purchase—if one can afford to—in order to feel more human. Consider the human need to have clear skies, to see trees and beautiful lanscapes, to feel connected with nature. Industrial urban life means smog, buildings on every horizon, and concrete pavements that insulate people from the earth. The aspiring young adult must inhabit this smoggy and unnatural environment if she or he wishes to become successful, but then after a certain modicum of success has been attained, she or he can begin to buy back what was given up, for instance, by moving to the suburbs or buying a home in the hills, thereby purchasing a clearer sky and a landscape with trees.

The therapist's fees, like the mortgage on a home in the hills, can be understood as a cost of rediscovering aspects of one's humanity that were set aside during the climb up the ladder of success. And the men's movement, like the psychotherapy industry, appeals to men who are relatively successful but unhappy. If the weekend gathering and telling of stories merely serves to satiate the average man's desire for brotherhood and meaning and he returns to his everyday life without creating anything new from what he learned, then men's gatherings will become simply an interesting diversion for an affluent minority of men. What if it turns out that the men who say they want to change the definition of masculinity merely want to feel better, to feel less constricted by the cruel requirements of the "real man" role? What is to keep men from using their privileges and power to develop new ways of being masculine without doing anything to end sexist gender relations?

The Political, Pro-Feminist Men's Movement

Among the ranks of the "political men," for instance, those who attend the annual National Conference on Men and Masculinity sponsored by the National Organization for Men Against Sexism (NOMAS), are men who teach gender studies at colleges, others who teach men who batter that there are better ways to live among women and children, activists in the struggle for gay and lesbian rights, activists in the struggle against AIDS, quite a few therapists and healers who do "men's work," and others who ascribe to the three prongs of the NOMAS program: "pro-feminist, gay affirmative, enhancing men's lives" (Laphan, 1990). The conferences are not huge—there were just under five hundred people at the sixteenth M&M conference in June, 1991 in Tucson—and occur only once a year. One large contingent of the men attending are straight, another gay and another bisexual. The dialogues are inspiring. Imagine gay and bisexual men, in a public forum, accusing straights of homophobia, and the straights listening very attentively in order to understand what the gays mean. The bisexual men also speak about their feeling that they "disappear" when men think in either/or terms about gay and straight.

Michael Kimmel (1991) offers a "pro-feminist" analysis of men's lives, and suggests a political strategy for the men's movement. He includes a struggle in the workplace to halt sexual harassment, a campaign to end date rape, and a collective assault on AIDS. It is a good program. Its enactment would help to change for the better what it means to be a man. A political perspective like Kimmel's, or like that of NOMAS provides the piece that is missing for me at other men's gatherings.

The problem with any political strategy that enumerates priority issues is that other deserving issues are necessarily excluded from the list. I would add to Kimmel's list the struggle to save workers' jobs in an age of workplace mechanization, speedup and runaway plants; and the struggle to save the schools and create meaningful work for inner city youth. Unemployment, underemployment and demeaning working conditions are the biggest cause of inadequacy in American men today. The gap is widening between the rich and the poor, and politicians of both parties are trying to convince the middle class that the only way they can solidify their position among the rich is by jettisoning the poor, ignoring the homeless, and locking lawbreakers in prison. The result is that twenty-five percent of young black males are incarcerated or on probation or parole. Instead of scratching our heads at men's events wondering why so few blue collar workers and men of color are in attendance, we could be reaching out and joining the struggles of working class and minority men to improve working and living conditions. In fact, many of the men who consider themselves political and attend men's events are doing just that—but it is difficult to reflect that kind of political commitment in a list of programmatic priorities. Likewise, the struggle to prevent war and nuclear annihilation should be high on the list of priorities for the men's movement. I am certain Kimmel and other list writers would agree.

The progressive, political sector of the men's movement faces a difficult challenge: given the dual potential of men's emerging awareness of gender issues, what can be done to push the movement in a progressive direction? For instance, there are some men who would channel the mushrooming men's movement into a campaign to increase men's rights, including the right to greater child visitation and the right not to be denied a job on account of affirmative action policies. At a time when women and gays are suffering from sexual harassment and gay-bashing and straight white men occupy an inordinate proportion of the positions of power in this inequitable society, I do not believe men's rights are the top priority. Men are needed in the struggle for abortion rights, the struggle to end men's violence against women, the struggle to attain equal opportunity for all at the workplace, the struggle to end sexual harassment and racism on the job, the struggle to end gay-bashing, and the list goes on. But in order to win support among men for the struggle to end gender inequity, political men must relate to what makes men dissatisfied with their lot and draws them to men's books and men's events.

Pro-feminist men risk becoming too one-sidedly political and losing sight of the psychological pain and spiritual vacuum that plagues so many men. Men who are hurting might not be interested in running to the aid of women who are oppressed, and this is especially the case if a man believes his immediate pain was caused by a woman's rejection. And a one-sided political analysis loses sight of the spiritual quest so many men are undertaking. As I mentioned in Chapter Four in relation to pornography, there is some danger that political, pro-feminist men will be viewed as self-righteous and judgmental, and will thereby lose many potential supporters for the anti-sexist men's movement.

Bob Connell's (1992) review of Robert Bly's *Iron John* and Sam Keen's *Fire in the Belly* suffers from this kind of one-sidedness. Connell pokes fun at the men who gather in the woods and beat drums. Then he suggests a political strategy that includes more men sharing in childrearing, struggling to end sexual harassment and other sexist and homophobic practices, working toward equal employment opportunities for women and gays, organizing political support for battered women's shelters and rape crisis centers, and so forth. It is a very good agenda for the men's movement. Again, one might add other items. The problem is that Connell sets up an us-versus-them dichotomy of political-versus-nonpolitical men, and then fails to offer the latter group any reason to ascribe to his political agenda if they do not already agree with his set of political principles. How can political men recruit those who have not yet made the connections? Certainly not by proclaiming that the "correct" political strategy is to fight for a particular list of things.

Connell ends his review by suggesting: "Maybe some of the warriors would care to come down from the hills and lend a hand in the cause of social justice." This is not a bad idea. But first, someone must prove to those warriors that by coming out of the hills and struggling to end sexism and other forms of domination, they will be improving their own lives in important ways. Perhaps they are afraid that in the new world of strong women, liberated gays, and pro-feminist men they would be forced to be serious and politically correct all of the time, and life would be a drag.

Men cannot be politicized by condemning all that it has meant to them to be a man. John Stoltenberg's (1989) *Refusing to Be a Man* errs in this direction. Men who feel some degree of dissatisfaction with the "real man" role and feel slightly inadequate, but refuse to compensate by resorting to sexism—just the men a political men's movement wants to attract—do not want to hear about refusing to be a man. They want reasons to feel good about who they are, including their masculine qualities. The men's movement must validate men's strengths—for instance their capacity to protect and provide for those they love—because men will never change if all they hear is that everything they have stood for until now is politically incorrect.

At the end of a lecture I gave on men's issues at the Berkeley Men's Center for Therapy in 1991 a man in the audience asked: "But don't men suffer as much or more than women?" The question was disconcerting because I had just finished arguing that men need to become more aware of the suffering of women at the hands of abusive men. I began my response by pointing out ways women are more oppressed, for instance the man who asked the question does not have to worry about being raped whenever he walks on the street at night. Then I caught myself. I was simply recapitulating the argument of my lecture while missing the underlying meaning of the man's question. This man was unhappy, he did not consider himself a sexist, and he would like someone, for a change, to pay attention to the roots of his unhappiness. I changed my tack. I said it is not a matter of who suffers more, rather it is about how gender relations based on domination are not good for anyone. The man was not quite happy with my answer, but others in the audience told me afterward that they were relieved that I had at least responded to his concern while not acceding to his suggestion that we forget about the women and concentrate exclusively on improving the plight of men.

A lesson of the 1960s was that you cannot organize people to sacrifice their own self-interests. A segment of the Students for a Democratic Society (SDS) campaigned on the slogan of giving up "white skin privileges." Very courageously aligning themselves with the poor and downtrodden, activists who ascribed to the principle of giving up privileges were buoyed for awhile by the large number of antiwar protesters who seemed to agree that white youth must give up certain privileges if all are to have equal opportunity. But then when the Viet Nam War ended and the self-interest of white college students was no longer served by taking to the streets to protest the draft, the mass movements waned. Activists' pleas to give up the privileges that derive from the oppression of others fell on deaf ears as a generation of rebels returned to relatively compliant lives.

Instead of asking men to give things up, including the little power they feel they have, the movement could attend to what ails men, and try to integrate their attempts to cure what ails them with a political struggle to end what, at its core, is wrong with our gendered social arrangements. There is only one way to accomplish this huge task: the political program of the men's movement must be responsive to men's needs while at the same time offering a larger vision. In other words, instead of telling men they must give away their power, we might turn our attention to helping men cross the lines that constrict their possibilities and redefine power in a way that makes it possible for men to feel powerful and yet not be sexist or homophobic. This is a tall order.

CHAPTER TEN

Crossing and Redrawing the Lines

Masculinity is all about the lines a man must not cross, and men do not stray very far outside the lines. I have mentioned some of the lines men draw in the sand, and how hard it is for us to cross them. For instance, how hard it is for men to let up on their steady pace, to jettison their arrhythmicity in order to take care of a sick parent or spend extra time with a child. There is a line that delineates acceptable male behaviors: men avoid dressing flamboyantly, stifle their feelings in public, do not hold hands or hug other men too openly, and in many other regards carefully avoid doing anything that might lead other men to think they are gay. Men try not to appear weak or dependent, and they do not back down.

Crossing lines can be lonely and disquieting. If a man crosses the line at work by valuing his family responsibilities more than he values rising in the hierarchy, he risks being stigmatized as "too sentimental," "not committed enough to the company," "not one of the guys." Men who are very involved with their children are considered losers in terms of career; men who are too responsive to a woman's needs are called "Momma's boys" or "soft males," and so forth. If we are to change traditional notions of masculinity for the better, we have quite a few lines to cross, and we will have to do something to change the way men are ostracized for crossing lines. We can begin by examining the ways lines are traditionally drawn.

Schoolyard Fights

I was not prepared for schoolyard fights. I had brothers, and we would fight. But there was an unwritten code at home that you never actually hit a brother, especially not in the face. So our fights were usually ninety percent wrestling, and when we did swing at each other we always made sure we missed. Somehow older brother taught the code to younger, even though no words were ever spoken.

In the third grade I was in an argument with another boy that led to some pushing and shouting. Suddenly, certainly without my ever expecting it, he swung and hit me in the face with his closed fist. I cried. I think some of the tears must have been on account of having to give up the reassuring illusion that all boys played by my family's unstated code. I learned the more universal code of the schoolyard, what Connell (1987, 1990) calls "hegemonic masculinity." Boys do not cry. Boys do not walk away from fights. And if you do either, you're chicken, a sissy, or queer.

After recovering from that incident, I, like all grade school boys, had to make a decision about how I would respond in the future when called to fight. I happened to be fairly strong, and with a certain amount of practice wrestling at home I could grab most boys my age and throw them to the ground. The problem was that other boys watching the tussle would not then consider the fight over, and did not consider me the victor. You had to punch the other guy. I, on the other hand, had not given up entirely on the original family code, nor did I particularly want to hurt anyone—or be hurt. So I could not bring myself to hit very hard. In two other memorable fights I threw my opponent to the ground, pinned his arm behind his back and tried to hurt him just enough to make him give up. He and the other boys would say I was unwilling to really fight. Some said I was chicken. And I think a kind of truce evolved, they feeling superior to me because I did not want to "really fight," me feeling a little safe knowing I could throw most of them to the ground and that few of them wanted that to happen. Even though this meant I had gained some respect from the other boys, I continued into adulthood to harbor a nagging suspicion that I might really be chicken. I discussed none of this with my brothers, of course, that would have been a violation of the family code.

It was not until I was in a leaderless men's group in my thirties that I finally felt safe enough, and sufficiently compelled, to relate my story about schoolyard fights. The group met for about five years in the late 1970s. At the end of one weekly meeting we agreed to discuss schoolyard fights at the following meeting. I remember the anxious anticipation. Would they consider me chicken? The evening came, we told our stories—some of the men had been fighters, some had avoided fights at all costs, one had "chickened out," and I believe one confessed having been a bully. But it did not matter. The men in the room listened attentively to every man's story, sympathized (we found out no one really liked the schoolyard scenario, not even the bully), and we all laughed about how serious it had seemed once.

My problem in grade school was that I was not yet sufficiently formed as an autonomous individual to fathom a tenable third alternative for myself. I did opt to do something other than slugging it out—wrestling my opponents to the ground—but, perhaps because I was unable to exude enough confidence in my alternative stance, the other boys were able to make me doubt my manliness. And boys who were having the same difficulty were unable to support each other at that time because all of us believed "real men" just did not do that sort of thing. Our shame depended on our social isolation. For most men, the idea that there is a tenable third alternative to the drama of top and bottom is a revelation that comes much later, the early years being dominated by the either/or theme.

Casualties of War

In *Casualties of War*, the 1989 film starring Michael J. Fox as Pfc. Erikson and Sean Penn as Sgt. Meserve, a patrol of five soldiers on a dangerous mission in Viet Nam kidnap a civilian woman from a neighboring village, gang rape, and murder her. The incident actually occurred, and the movie illustrates well what I mean by crossing lines. War, like prison, makes men's issues stand out in boldface. There is Sgt. Meserve, the "real man" who fights heroically, protects and takes care of his men, and feels that because he was not permitted by his C.O. to visit a whorehouse the night before, he is "entitled" to steal a "girl" from the village and use her for his sadistic sexual pleasure and then discard the body. Then there is Pfc. Erikson, who is forced to stand by and watch the rape and murder. At first Sgt. Meserve and the others try desparately to convince Erikson to join them in their "sexual fun." Taunts are thrown Erikson's way, taunts that contain a menacing threat of violence. One man yells: "Erikson doesn't want to ball the chick!" Another says: "Maybe he's a queer." Another chimes in: "He's a chickenshit!" When it becomes clear Erikson will not change his mind and join the others, Sgt. Meserve glares at him and threatens: "Maybe when I'm done with her I'm going to take my turn with you!" Another soldier, Diaz, had declared to Erikson he did not want any part in the rape. Meserve, sensing the potential alliance between Diaz and Erikson, jokes about the possibility of the two of them having a homosexual affair. Thus Erikson and Diaz are intimidated so that they will not adopt a third, alternative stance in regard to the male culture of the patrol that requires one to participate in gang rape in order to be "one of the guys." Diaz does change his mind and joins in the gang rape.

The requirements for membership among the "real men" are established and the outsider, Erikson, is called "chickenshit" and "queer" and threatened with sodomy. It takes much courage for a man to cross the line that "real men" draw in the sand in order to follow the dictates of his own conscience, just as in the workplace it takes courage for a male worker to refuse to take part in the daily sexual harassment that goes on in the name of "good clean fun." Michael J. Fox's character crosses the line by empathizing with the woman, by refusing to be "one of the guys" and participating in the defiling of a woman, and finally he reports the incident, breaking the most important rule: "real men don't snitch."

Pfc. Erikson goes up the line of command, telling two officers about the incident, and each responds that he should forget about it. Finally, a chaplain listens to his story and initiates an investigation. The soldiers involved attempt to kill Erikson in retaliation. The movie ends with Pfc. Erikson back home suffering from symptoms of posttraumatic stress disorder as well as the perpetual dread that one of the soldiers he reported will be released from prison and come after him seeking revenge.

Sex Roles

The lines across which men do not cross seem well defined, yet difficult to describe. Most men believe certain things are expected of them "as men," and yet, when asked to delineate those expectations, men get flustered and protest they cannot really come up with a list—and then when men do produce their lists no two men agree on the items to include. But all men agree on one thing: traditional sex roles are constricting.

Just as men cannot agree on the list of expectations that go with the male role, there is little agreement among scholars on the theoretical model that best describes men's experience. The current debate focuses on "role theory," which has held sway in departments of sociology since Talcott Parsons (Parsons & Bales, 1955) explicated the basics. We are socialized to play roles in society. For instance, gender-appropriate behaviors and attitudes are taught to young children. Thus there are proper or "normal" roles for men as well as for women—Parsons offers that famous dichotomy: men are "instrumental" while women are "expressive"—and men as well as women learn their parts in the course of socialization. Anyone who does not play their gendered part well is subject to stigmatization as a deviant.

There are a number of critiques of role theory. Joseph Pleck (1981) charges that role theorists clump all men into a homogeneous population as if all were trying to play the same role, thus failing to explain the diversity among men and the variety of "role models." In addition, if there is a clear masculine role and any man who fails to play the correct role is stigmatized, how does one explain the changing social functions of men and the evolving forms of masculinity? For instance, Barbara Ehrenreich (1983) traces the evolution of middle class male roles from the 1950s through the 1980s: In the 1950s there was the conformist, the man in the grey flannel suit who worked hard and was a good provider; then there were the noncomformists, the playboys of Hugh Hefner's generation, the beatniks, the humanistic psychologists, and the androgynous hippies in revolt against conformism; and then, with the women's movement, there was the evolution of new roles for both sexes and a "male revolt" against the "breadwinner ethic." Role theory is unable to explain these developments.

The omnipresence of institutional racism in our society sets up very different roles for black men (the same is true for other minorities as well as for different classes). According to Clyde Franklin (1987), because of the "institutional decimation" of black men that is reflected in the fact that so many grow up in poverty, land in prison, or are murdered at an early age, young black male sex-role expectations include toughness, sexual conquest, and thrill seeking—all of which serve to mitigate the low self-esteem that results from racism and the black male's inability to satisfy traditional majority male role expectations.

Arthur Brittan (1989) is critical of role theory as well as psychoanalysis to the extent that these "mechanical" approaches assign abstract qualities to each gender and assume these qualities are fixed at a very early stage of socialization.

> But what if we argued to the contrary, namely that gender identity is infinitely negotiable, that the specification of masculine and feminine traits was simply an aspect of a continuing process of interactive relationships in which both men and women mutually construct, confirm, reject or deny their identity claims? Why should we assume that identity is predetermined or made in the crucible of family relationships? (p. 35)

And Michael Kimmel (1987) argues that role theory minimizes the way male and female roles are mutually determinative, and ignores the importance of power in gender relations.

In order to transcend these deficiencies in sex-role theory, Pleck (1981) would have us replace the sex-role paradigm with a "Sex-Role Strain Paradigm." He lists and contrasts the basic assumptions of the two paradigms. Sex-role theory holds that there is a male sex type: males learn their roles from identification with fathers and other men; the development of appropriate sex-role identity is a risky and failure-prone process; psychological health depends on the acquisition of an appropriate sex-type identity; homosexuality reflects a disturbance of sex-role identity; and problems in the area of sex-role identity are the cause of men's problems relating to women. In contrast, the sex-role strain paradigm contains a very different set of basic assumptions: sex roles are defined in relation to stereotypes; sex roles are contradictory and inconsistent (for instance, male adolescents are encouraged to excel in physical contests but as adults men are rewarded more for their intellectual prowess); a high proportion of men violate sex-role expectations and are condemned for it; fear of condemnation causes some men to overconform to the stereotypic roles; most men experience sex-role strain; and historical changes—for instance the "crisis in masculinity" we are now witnessing—cause sex-role strain. Pleck believes that the role-strain paradigm is much more adequate for the job of explaining historical changes in gender relations.

According to Bob Connell (1987), all role theories, including the role-strain paradigm, fall short in explaining gendered experience. He argues:

> Change is always something that happens to sex roles, that impinges on them—whether from the direction of the society at large (as in discussions of how technological and economic change demands a shift to a "modern" male sex role) or from the direction of the asocial "real self" inside the person, demanding more room to breathe. Sex-role theory cannot grasp change as a dialectic arising within gender relations themselves. (pp. 78–79)

He also points out that role theory fails to attend to domination and ways it might be transcended. Connell is critical of Pleck's role-strain paradigm as well. For instance, he claims Pleck's paradigm rests on "the fixed dichotomy of sex," and is concerned only with "mapping changes in attitudes and expectations about the dichotomy." Connell would have us radically alter the dichotomy itself. I will not pursue the academic debate any further, the reader who is interested in the details can turn to the voluminous literature, beginning with the work of Pleck, Connell, Kimmel, and Brittan.

The mystifications of theory reflect those in the real social world, in this case one might say that men-on-the-street are as confused as the academics about their roles, and they think in static terms about the male role because they cannot imagine things ever being very different. Most men think in terms of a "right way" for men to do things, and even though there would be little if any consensus among men regarding the specifics of that "right" male way, most men believe that when their lives begin to go awry it is a sign of their inadequacy as men. While role theory attempts to delineate the "right way," it provides no place for an alternative vision.

Connell (1987, 1990) points out that global dominance of men over women results in, and is legitimized by, a narrowing and stereotyping of "hegemonic masculinity." According to Connell: "There is no femininity that is hegemonic in the sense that the dominant form of masculinity is hegemonic among men" (p. 183). Other forms of masculinity, like homosexuality, are subordinated to the dominant stereotype, despite the fact that "the cultural ideal (or ideals) of masculinity need not correspond at all closely to the actual personalities of the majority of men" (p. 184). All men share a stereotype of the "real man" just as they share the male theme of top dog and fallen subordinate—the "real man" is the guy at the top of the hierarchy. Most men feel inadequate relative to that standard, yet the majority of men do not even aspire to become that stereotype! For instance, many men abhor the way corporate executives, public administrators, and politicians abuse power and mistreat underlings; yet these same men feel inadequate because they wield very little power in the public arena and are unable to manipulate institutions in the interest of improving their lives and the lives of their intimates. The discrepancy between the stereotype of the dominant male and the actuality of most men's lives serves to maintain a sense of inadequacy in most men and to support the social pattern of male dominance. Blye Frank (1987) underscores the importance of homophobia in the maintenance of gender dominance by suggesting the term "hegemonic heterosexual masculinity."

According to Connell (1987), masculinity takes a variety of forms.

Their interrelation is centered on a single structural fact, the global dominance of men over women. This structural fact provides the main basis for relationships among men that define a hegemonic form of masculinity in the society as a whole. "Hegemonic masculinity" is always constructed in relation to various subordinated masculinities as well as in relation to women. The interplay between different forms of masculinity is an important part of how a patriarchal social order works. (p. 183)

It is the "hegemony" of a dominant notion of masculinity—in the media, in the rules for schoolyard fights, and in the boardroom—that prevents men from exploring the possibility there might be something very wrong with the way our sex roles are written and our social relations are arranged.

This does not mean we should seek a single, correct alternative version of masculinity. Harry Brod (1987) comments:

> The level of somewhat sweeping generalizations attests to men's studies still being in its infancy (as many of these authors would be the first to admit), as does the widespread tendency to speak in the singular of the male sex role rather than different modes of masculinity that vary by race, class, ethnicity, sexual orientation, nationality, and so on. (pp. 50–51)

The implication of Brod's work is that we can strive to increase tolerance for a variety of roles for men, and no man should be stigmatized for not playing any particular one.

Role theory is just one of many possible ways to explain how lines are drawn across which "real men" do not tread. What is needed is not the single abstract theory or "correct" explanation of the way the lines are drawn, rather we need to understand what makes men hesitate to cross, to collectively redraw the lines that constrict, and to do all this with a strong sense of brotherhood and power. Stigmatization is an obstacle for men who would cross and redraw the lines. While sociologists speak of deviance, clinicians speak of psychopathology. Both involve the stigmatization of those who would cross the lines that circumscribe traditional ways of being and doing.

Gender and Psychopathology

In psychotherapy, it is often important to distinguish between the client's idiosyncratic psychopathology—his inner flaws—and the qualities and dilemmas that he shares with most men. A male client tells me he has no friends, and wonders why he is having so much difficulty finding men he really likes. We explore his psychological issues, including the intense childhood rivalry he experienced with his brothers, and the way his father, who played favorites among the boys, rewarded him for "one-upping and never trusting the others." This psychological insight is useful, and he quickly sees how it can be applied in his current dilemma. For instance, he can reexamine the issue of trust and attempt to keep the ghost of his boyhood father out of his current relationships with males. But then he still has to transcend the gender-specific foibles that he shares with so many men, the ways male posturing prevents us from finding more meaningful ways to relate. Aware of his own personally driven need to continue the pattern of male distancing and posturing, he is at least in better position to struggle with other men to achieve the kind of friendship and intimacy he craves.

Gender and psychopathology are intricately linked. Clinicians tend to think about gender roles in terms of psychopathology. Freud tended to diagnose pathology in places where he found deviance from Victorian gender expectations, for instance, ambition in women or homosexuality. (Exceptions occurred when Freud did not agree with popular views about gender. For instance, he accepted women students and treated quite a few as peers at a time when society expected women to stay home and rear children.) He believed that men who lacked a "normal" supply of male ambition were unconsciously surrendering to their castrating fathers, and that women who tried too hard to succeed in the traditionally male world were suffering from penis envy. In other words, men and women who cross certain lines are told they suffer from psychopathology. Several psychoanalysts have taken Freud to task for his theory of gender and deviance (Horney, 1924, 1926, 1935; Jones, 1927; Mitchell, 1974; Thompson, 1942, 1943; Weisstein, 1970; Zilboorg, 1944).

Phyllis Chesler (1976) presents other examples from the history of psychiatry where women are deemed insane because they refuse to play the prescribed female role, including the case of Elizabeth Packard (1816–c. 1890), who was locked up in an asylum for many years merely because her husband, enraged at her refusal to bow to his authority, declared her insane; the law gave him the prerogative to have his wife committed while she had no equivalent right. I have illustrated gender bias in the construction of categories of mental illness in the case of late luteal phase dysphoric disorder. Why are women's cycles pathologized while men's compulsive need to maintain a steady pace is not? Of course, the reason is that the male proclivity to override natural cycles fits the needs of our competitive, bureaucratic public world.

The lines are not yet rigidly drawn. There is still room for debate in the American Psychiatric Association about the inclusion of premenstrual syndrome (PMS) among the list of official forms of mental disease, and the APA modified that list in 1973 when gay and lesbian activists were able to convince the membership that homosexuality is not an illness. But the fact remains that the lines are being drawn in the process of establishing a classification of mental disorders. In other words, when a behavior or attitude is deemed to lie beyond the line it is described as a symptom of a specific pathological condition.

The interplay of roles and psychopathology becomes quite obvious in the case of the person deemed mad. Sociologists of deviance—including Erving Goffman (1961) and Thomas Scheff (1966)—argue that certain people in society are labelled "mentally ill," and that labelling initiates a social process of behavior-shaping that consolidates their role as deviants while also serving to maintain the social equilibrium, since these deviants mark by their excesses the boundaries of normal behavior. The "treatment" reserved for the mentally ill and other deviants—including stigmatization, incarceration, involuntary medication, and, in many cases, dreadful inattention to basic human needs—serve as a warning to those who would veer off the "normal" path.

In fact, the lines that separate normalcy from mental illness resemble the lines that create our definition of manliness, even though they are drawn in different places and there are different things one must do in order to be considered deviant. Thus, if one takes off one's clothes in public one is likely to be deemed mad, while it is the wearing of unusual clothes—especially clothes that are associated with women or gays—that results in one being deemed unmanly or effeminate. The lines that are drawn by our current understanding of psychopathology, like the lines that circumscribe the "real man" role, constrict our range. It is because a large number of men are no longer willing to suffer the constriction that there is so much interest in "men's issues" today.

At this stage of the incipient men's movement a large number of men are visiting psychotherapists and asking for guidance on the unfamiliar path ahead. Of course, for psychotherapists, a thorough knowledge of psychopathology is what informs therapeutic interventions and strategies. As was explained in Chapter Nine, there is a dual potential here. To the extent men who step out of traditional gender expectations (or cross the line) are told they are suffering from some form of psychopathology, therapy serves to police the boundaries of traditional masculinity and slow men's progress in creating new definitions of manliness. Yet, if there could be a different relationship, for instance, if therapists could support the desire in their male clients to transcend traditional forms of masculinity, then therapy would be a valuable asset in the struggle to restructure gender roles and relations. Recent volumes on men in therapy, including *Men in Transition*, edited by Solomon and Levy (1982), and *Men in Therapy*, edited by Meth and

Pasick (1990), offer a ray of hope. No longer does phallocentrism have to reign in psychodynamic theorizing.

In this regard, the work of Jean Baker Miller (1976, 1988), Judith Jordan (1989), Stephen Bergman (1991), and their collaborators at the Stone Center of Wellesley College is promising. They believe that this culture's over-valuation of autonomy and independence leaves something to be desired in terms of community and the capacity to be intimate, and that a very male notion of independence and autonomy is at the core of traditional clinical descriptions of psychopathology. Thus, women are pathologized because of their emphasis on connection and interdependence. They call upon psychotherapists to tease out this unstated assumption and redraw the line between psychopathology and mental health so that women's need for connection and community will be viewed as an admirable trait rather than a symptom (Jordan, Kaplan, Miller, Stiver, & Surrey, 1991).

Crossing the Lines

If gender is socially constructed, there is room for change. That is cause for hope for a men's movement that would redefine male roles while ending some of the injustice and inhumanity that prevail in our competitive, narcissistic culture today. But our entrapment within traditional notions of gender—whether we talk about this in terms of gender roles or in terms of normal versus pathological behavior—keeps us from seeing the potential for change. Given the hegemony of traditional masculinity, the tendency for men to stigmatize noncom- forming men and the tendency for men to be isolated and unconnected with each other, the crossing of certain lines requires great courage.

Artists light the path by imagining a very different reality (Marcuse, 1978). Sometimes it is as much the way they live as it is their work. For instance, I believe Vaclav Havel (1990), then President of Czechoslovakia, made a powerful statement about traditional male roles in the speech he gave when he was awarded an honorary degree at the Hebrew University in Jerusalem. He confessed he suffered from feelings of unworthiness and, like a Kafka character, he could easily imagine being taken by the scruff of his neck and thrown out of the hall. He told his esteemed audience:

> You may well ask how someone who thinks of himself this way can be the president of a country. It's a paradox, but I must admit that if I am a better president than many others would be in my place, then it is precisely because somewhere in the deepest substratum of

my work lies this constant doubt about myself and my right to hold office.

As I began reading Havel's speech I assumed he would proceed from a declaration of his unworthiness to an uplifting point, perhaps about the history and fate of Eastern Europe. But he continued to speak of his own unworthiness, ending with these words:

> Once more, I thank you for the honor, and after what I've said here, I'm ashamed to repeat that I accept it with a sense of shame."

What a brilliant performance! Instead of posturing as world leaders do, he admits he feels small in the face of the overwhelming international problems that confront all of us.

Havel's humility comes to mind as I listen to a client tell me about his shame. Phil, a gay man in his mid-forties, tells me about a small dinner party with several friends. At one point he was speaking for several minutes in an excited tone when one of his friends loudly told him to shut up so others can have a chance to talk. He felt "mortified." He ceased talking immediately, remained silent for the remainder of the evening, and felt depressed for several days. We discussed his ambivalence about being spontaneous and effusive, and his fear that his exuberance would lead to humiliation. He recalled that in his family he was expected to smile politely, "be nice," and avoid displays of excitement and intense emotionality. As a child it was easy for him to suppress his exuberance, but he was less able to disguise the moments of pain and sadness behind a smiling face. I asked what happened when he displayed unhappy feelings in this family of happy faces, and he revealed that his parents and siblings tended to poke fun at him for being so sensitive. This exhange led to the topic of shame. He told me he felt "shamed" at the dinner and that his friend's criticism "knocked the wind out of my sails."

Phil is ashamed of his emotional range. His mood swings are not wide enough to warrant a clinical diagnosis of manic-depressive disorder or even cyclothymic personality, but they do draw notice and condemnation from his family. As an adult he is easily shamed and lacks resilience to weather the strains in social situations. His personal foibles mirror the social dilemma of men whose emotional range is beyond that permitted by traditional male roles. Unlike Havel, whose performance becomes a public statement about the limitations of traditional male posturing, Phil feels shame whenever his effusiveness runs counter to what is deemed appropriate behavior. He does not have a hard time talking to women; his women friends never complain about his effusiveness. We talk about gender roles and the constrictions tradition places on men's range of expressiveness, and we compare it to his family's requirement that he be a "nice guy" and know his place. He decides to phone the friend who cut him off at the dinner and tell him he is angry at him for being so intolerant and cruel. This action will not change his situation drastically, but at least he is beginning to transcend his shame and isolation.

Phil is not alone. Shame prevents men from crossing lines and redefining masculinity (Osherson, 1992). Each man has a personal story to tell. Many compensate for their shame with workaholism, abuse of women, alcohol and drugs, and other self-destructive and isolating patterns. When Phil and I talk about his shame and link it with the issue of gender and the limitations of the traditional male role, he is able to get past his personal hell and do something to alter the interpersonal situation that sent him into a depression. Havel's leadership is reflected in his ability to display personal foibles in public and make a political statement that calls on all of us to reconsider our assumptions about what constitutes leadership and manliness. Shame develops where there is isolation; the shamed child goes to his room rather than seeking company and support. The sharing of the roots of our shame and the collective reexamination of our underlying assumptions provide an opportunity for us to reverse the pattern, to transcend shame while redefining masculinity.

There are many other ways to cross the lines that constrict men's lives. We cross the lines when we walk down the street holding hands. We cross the lines when we tell the boss at work we cannot stay late because we have childrearing responsibilities. We cross the lines when we refuse to laugh at a sexist affront against a female colleague, homophobic slanders against gay workmates, and other episodes of sexual harassment at the workplace. We do it independently, as conscious men who are committed to ending sexism and homophobia. But it is much easier to cross the lines when one has supporters—a partner who shares one's views, friends who listen to the problems one encounters crossing the line at work, and others who are actively struggling to improve gender relations.

I have discovered that men's difficulties being intimate—with other men as well as with women—make it more difficult to cross and redraw the lines. Miller (1983), at the beginning of his study of men's friendships, told a friend what he wanted to do, only to have the friend warn:

Male friendship. You mean you're going to write about homosexuality. That's what everybody will think, at least. Could be
dangerous for you. (p. 2)

There is a vicious cycle that makes it very difficult for men who would
change: if one is to cross the lines that define traditional masculinity
and thereby risk being stigmatized and devalued, one needs the support
of other men, but men tend to distance themselves from a man who
seems different or unmanly, so the crossing tends to be very lonely.
This is why improving our intimacies with each other and evolving
better support networks are such important tasks for men who would
take risks and cross the lines that constrict our possibilities.

Friendship could be the key to breaking the vicious cycle. But the
difficulties men have being friends are aggravated by the cyclic
dynamic. For instance, men are socialized to believe one can judge a
man's worth in relation to the men he befriends. In school it is a matter
of having friends who are popular, athletic, smart, stylish, sufficiently
rebellious, or otherwise part of an in-crowd. Later in life, it is a matter
of having friends who are successful, well-connected, sufficiently
sophisticated or interesting, of the right class or demeanor, and
otherwise unlikely to be an embarassment. Association with gays,
losers, or "unmanly" friends can be the undoing of a man who is trying
to achieve status in the hierarchy. But who are the men who take the
lead in redefining gender? They tend to be soft-spoken, in touch with
the feminine if not gay, uninterested in the usual male pursuits, and
"too" interested in raising a family and working on relationships with
partners and friends. It is time to ask on what basis the lines are drawn,
and to begin redrawing them.

Soft Males and Mama's Boys

The evolving men's movement, even while refusing to support a
traditional notion of the "real man," is beginning to construct
hierarchies and categories of deviance of its own. For instance, in parts
of the new men's movement there is intolerance of "softness" in men.
The basic idea is that certain men are Mama's boys or "pussy whipped,"
meaning they were too tied to their mothers as children, and as adults
they are too tender, too empathic, too interested in women's issues. But
against what standard is this "too" measured? Of course, the standard is
a new version of the familiar concept of a "real man." The traditional
concept is that a "real man" is strong, brave, independent, relatively
unemotional, unflinching, *and properly distanced from the female*

perspective and from identification with women. The new concept, more acceptable to sensitive men, is that a "real man" gathers with other men, tells his story, talks about feelings, plays drums, takes part in primitive dances and rituals, *and is properly distanced from the female perspective and from identification with women.*

Robert Bly's (1982, 1990) notion of "soft males" reflects and encourages this stigmatization. Bly suggests there is a step beyond feminism men must take. He begins by describing the "soft males" of the 'seventies:

> They're lovely, valuable people—I like them—they're not inter-
> ested in harming the earth or starting wars. There's a gentle
> attitude toward life in their whole being and style of living. But
> many of these men are not happy. You quickly notice the lack of
> energy in them. They are life-preserving but not exactly *life-giving.*
> Ironically, you often see these men with strong women who
> positively radiate energy. (1990, pp. 2–3)

Bly believes that the man who wishes to be liberated from the bonds of the traditional male image must traverse two further stages of adult development: first he must get in touch with his feminine side, his "interior woman," and second he must get in touch with the wildman inside him, the "deep male." In order to accomplish the second step, the man must resolve certain issues with his father, and go to other men for help finding his way. The male who is attuned to the issue of gender equality has traversed the first stage but not the second. I agree with Bly there is another step men must take, and I agree that men must talk to other men about this, not just to women. But I do not think it is merely a matter of distancing women and getting in touch with the "wild man" within, the source of life and power that has been repressed in the "soft male."

In Bly's (1990) telling of the story of Iron John, the wild man in Grimm's fairy tale who is captured in the forest and locked in a cage in the center of town, a boy is playing with a golden ball, the ball roles into the cage and the wild man grabs it. The boy asks him to return it and he refuses—unless the boy will free him from the cage. The boy protests he does not have the key. The wild man retorts that the key is under his mother's pillow. In other words, if the boy is to get in touch with the wild man deep within, with his desires and his power, he must break free of his mother. There is a truth to discover in the story, of course.

The problem is that Bly goes too far in the direction of blaming and devaluing women when he repeatedly accuses mothers of smothering sons. In Bly's writings and public lectures women are rarely mentioned, and when they are the most frequent comment is that mothers smother their sons. He rarely mentions the mother's role in nurturing and raising the son. Juxtaposing this observation with Bly's emphasis on forgiving the errant father, it seems fair to conclude there is a significant bias against women and against dependency on women.

Then, when asked by Bill Moyers in a television interview if the phenomenon of men's gatherings in the 1980s and 1990s is not an outgrowth of the women's movement of the 1960s and 1970s, Bly makes light of Moyers' suggestion and insists the men's movement developed independently of the women's. It is as if he is so concerned lest his masculinity seem reactive to women that he has to devalue women and refuse to acknowledge their contribution to the evolution of a heightened gender consciousness. Meanwhile, he rarely mentions the fact that men oppress women and says nothing about the need for men and women to join in the struggle to put an end to sexism. In fact, in the Moyers interview, he says that women are unhappy mainly because they, like men, did not get enough of their fathers' attention. What about sexual oppression, exclusion from positions of power, unequal pay, rape, and other forms of sexual oppression? Bly is silent.

There is some danger that men might move on from the stage of supporting women's struggles to evolve a new, more "sensitive" and "spiritual" form of sexism. For instance, with so much focus on avoiding passivity and feeling powerful, too little attention is given to the need for men to admit to weakness, painful emotions, and dependency needs, and to develop the capacity to tolerate these qualities in others and to nurture.

In addition, Bly practically ignores the experience of gay men (the exception is a token reference in the introduction to *Iron John*). Gordon Murray (1991) points out that Bly speaks of Apollo and Hyacinthus without mentioning that they were lovers, and describes in some detail the tribal initiation rites in Papua New Guinea while carefully avoiding mention of the fact that the older men pass their semen to young male initiates (Lidz & Lidz, 1986). Murray asks: "Why does he pick and choose from the mythological and tribal data, excluding references to homosexuality? I think it's Bly's homophobia. It's a type common among liberals of his generation, a homophobia by making-invisible."

I was in a leaderless men's group for five years in the 1970s at the beginning of what is now called the men's movement, and I readily admit the group I was in and many others like it were formed by men who had a deep respect for the women who were demanding their rights. We not only did not want to be left out, but also we believed we had much to learn from the women's precedent—and we struggled to evolve ways to transcend the male posturing that had kept us apart and isolated us until that time. Men's groups of that era typically began with discussions of men's problems relating to women. The successful groups eventually turned to the problems men have relating to each other, and solutions to those problems often led to improved relationships with women as well. Many of the men at gatherings I have attended come from similar backgrounds, or attend men's events because the women in their lives encourage them to do something about their alienation from their own inner life and from other men.

Let us assume for a moment that the women's movement is generally correct, and a large part of what ails our society is uncontrolled male posturing; for instance, men cannot back down from a fight, not on the street, not in the competitive world of business, and not in the international arena where they regularly challenge each other to wars where many thousands die. And let us assume for a moment that what is needed is more contact with "the feminine." The popular notion of "the feminine" currently includes the capacity to nurture and care about the fate of others, to respect and protect natural resources including our bodies and our rain forests, to be open about feelings and include feelings in our decision-making process, and so forth. Of course, there is also the "shadow" feminine—the evil witch, the envious mother—but in general, when one speaks of "the feminine" in men as well as in women, since Jung, the reference is to cooperation, nurturing, connectedness, respect for nature, and so forth.

Of course, as soon as I contrast masculine and feminine qualities I am relying on stereotypes, and these imply fixed, universal qualities for each category, and assume little diversity within categories. Stereotypes create an image of a large group of people—a gender, a nationality, a race, a sexual preference—and then all the members of that group are placed in the same cubbyhole, thus denying each his or her individuality and making it unlikely we will ever really get to know any member of that group. Stereotypes keep people apart, and once one group of people are distanced in this way from another there is fertile soil for projection and devaluation, as in the case of homophobia.

It should be quite clear to the reader by now that I believe there is nothing "natural" about the assignment of certain qualities and capacities to women. I do not believe that all women display the qualities I mentioned, nor that all men lack them. Still, the stereotypes reflect an aspect of reality. "Male" proclivities—including competition, concern about status in hierarchies, isolation, obsessional steadiness of pace and the use of women to enlarge one's ego—have led to our current political predicament; and a shift in the balance so that there is more "feminine" energy does seem a part of the antidote. I believe that, if we want to change our social priorities, not only must we shift the balance of energies in the direction we now stereotypically conceive of as "feminine," but we must also transcend the stereotypes in the process.

In this context, calling men Mama's boys, soft males, and pussy-whipped because they listen too much to women is quite counterproductive—the wrong male qualities are being stigmatized. It is precisely the men who admit to the strong influence of women—the men who do not feel a strong need to "dis-identify" with women at every opportunity—who can contribute most to changing gender relations. According to Bob Blauner (1991):

> Men in the movement are likely to have grown up closer to their mothers than to their fathers. Therefore there are a sizable number of "Mama's Boys," and the denial of this reality contributes to the movements's flight from mother—this is because we accept the male prescription and want to fulfill the criteria of adequacy in the new men's movement. (p. 28)

Bly leads us down a false path when he stigmatizes feminine qualities in men; at the same time, he has a point. What does he mean by "soft men?" On the one hand, he seems to be referring to men who have a highly developed feminine side, who have a deep respect for women and their power, who prefer connectedness and nurturing over combat and competition, and who eschew traditional male pursuits that involve cruelty, misogyny and homophobia. To the extent Bly devalues these qualities in men, he is leading us down a false path. On the other hand, he seems to be referring to men who are passive, unformed as individuals, entirely reactive to others' wishes and demands, and so frightened of anger and combat that they tend to back down and disavow what they stand for in the face of strong opposition. Here is where Bly has a point, this kind of "softness" is very limiting. Sam Keen (1991) offers an alternative to this kind of softness: "The historical challenge for modern men is clear—to discover a peaceful form of virility and to create an ecological commonwealth, to become fierce gentlemen" (p. 121).

But why should we apply the point exclusively to men? Women who are passive, unformed as individuals, entirely reactive, and afraid of their anger and strength are also quite limited human beings. This kind of "softness" is not good for either gender. When Bly links "softness" in men with excessive or prolonged connection to women, he makes two errors. First, he stigmatizes certain feminine, nurturing qualities in men. And second, he assumes that passivity and an inability to stand up for oneself are only problematic in men. In other words, it is more acceptable for women to be passive and not entirely formed as human beings.

There is another way that Bly's link between closeness with women and softness in men misses the mark. Bly implies that, if men would stop being "soft," they would stand up to the women who have gained so much power in recent years, and doing so would make men feel powerful again. This message appeals to many men who feel inadequate while they perceive women gaining power in our society. But this is a message of backlash (Faludi, 1991). The reason men feel powerless and inadequate is not that women have taken their power away. Shifts in the economy, high unemployment, plant closures and massive layoffs, higher taxes for the middle and lower classes with fewer social services, racism, a crisis in health care, inflated insurance premiums and other unfortunate social developments over the last fifteen years have made it more difficult for men to feel adequate and powerful. Bly allies with ultraconservative forces when he blames the plight of the American male on the emergence of powerful women in the public arena.

Finally, Bly's use of the term "soft" reflects another underlying assumption: that men's ways are strong and powerful while women's ways are "softer" and powerless. I do not accept that assumption! Cooperation, concern about the plight of others, respect for nature, and a host of other qualities we associate with women today are the ingredients for a greater power than men now have. For instance there is the power to make the personal political, the power to save the environment by rationally disposing of our waste products, and the power to avert nuclear annihilation.

I have discussed the need for men to stand up to the women in their lives in order to be able to resolve some of the tensions that regularly arise in heterosexual couples, and sometimes men must work through unresolved conflicts regarding their mothers in order to develop their capacity to stand toe-to-toe with women as adults. But this is not the same as saying women are to blame for men's feelings of inadequacy. If there is to be social progress, men and women must stand together against the wrongs of a patriarchal culture. Otherwise, power would be left to those who are more competitive, greedy, and ruthless. Men and women must be anything but "soft" (in the sense of passive, reactive, and unwilling to stand up for their interests) if we are to redraw the lines that constrict gendered behavior. But the toughness that is required will not come from stigmatizing men who are deeply connected with women and the feminine within.

Redrawing the Lines: Envisioning Different Gender Relations

I have described some of the lines we are constantly drawing, for instance the lines that delineate sex roles and psychopathology. I have pointed out that we too seldom examine the assumptions underlying the drawing of those lines, for instance, the assumption that the emotional cycles of women are pathological while the almost obsessive steadiness of men is normal even if it causes ulcers and heart attacks. It is time to consider another question: On what model do we think through the lines we deem worth crossing? In other words, if we were to be given the responsibility of rewriting the roles, redesigning the categories of psychopathology, and redefining masculinity, what normative standard would we employ in drawing new lines?

Some might protest at this point that no standard is acceptable, that as soon as we create a new standard there will be a new stigmatization. I believe there will always be deviants, no matter how progressive one's viewpoint—for instance, I will always consider racism and sexism to be undesirable deviations from proper human pursuits—but the things one stigmatizes reflect the vision one has for society. The reason I am concerned about the tendency in the men's movement to stigmatize softness and connection with mother is that the stigmatization contradicts my vision of a gender-equitable society. I do not believe it is possible to practice psychotherapy or to write about gender without having a normative model in mind. Since there will always be a process of socialization and there will always be qualities that we stigmatize, it is far better to be aware of the biases inherent in our implicit normative models than to deny there are any implicit norms in our judgments and thus become blind to our biases.

I certainly do not mean to imply we should cross all lines, nor that breaking barriers, or doing the unexpected, is always the thing to do. The result would be anarchy, chaos, and confusion. Nor do I mean we will eventually construct one proper form of masculinity; Brod's (1987) notion of a multiplicity of masculinities coexisting in an atmosphere of tolerance can be part of the redrawing. Rather, I am using the image of crossing lines as a metaphor to describe the constrictions that dwell in our gendered sensibility. The metaphor should not be taken too literally. We need to consider the merit of crossing those lines in one spot or another, and then we need to move on to the difficult task of collectively redrawing the lines. We will not always agree.

I propose we proceed by first envisioning a better society, and then extrapolating backward from that vision in order to decide which qualities in men we would like to reinforce and which we would like to change. Cooperation and concern about others are high on the list for reinforcement; racism, the urge to rape, and brutality are on the list for extinction. There is less consensus on other items; consider the debate on pornography. This is not a new idea—progressive social theorists have been utilizing this logic since Marx and the early socialists engaged in debates about values and politics. Imagine a Utopia or a better society, figure out what qualities would help to build such a place, and then begin to encourage the development of those qualities now, among ourselves and our children.

Women have had to take the lead here. Men, like the Master in Hegel's Master/Slave dialectic, know something is wrong and things must change, but are ambivalent about giving up their dominant status in order to bring about change. Attributing their current pains and discontents to losses in status they have suffered in recent times—for instance, because women have become too powerful—men yearn for the good old days when "a man was a man, a woman a woman, and they both knew their places." I have given several examples of ways in which traditional psychiatry, because of its inclination to voice male ideas and maintain men in power, reinforces yesterday's gender norms by diagnosing pathology whenever men or women fail to satisfy society's traditional roles and expectations. The best example is Freud's theory of penis envy.

Women, like Hegel's Slave, are not only willing and eager to give up their subordinate status, but also are compelled by their situation to see precisely what the Master has a very hard time seeing; that only by ending domination can anyone hope to be free. Because of the way their oppression as women unites their gender, and because they have only oppression to look back on, women are compelled to move forward collectively. Where male psychiatry traditionally looks backward in establishing models of normal gender behavior, women and gays are redrawing the lines and redirecting the therapeutic process to prepare people to cope in a better world, for instance, a world where men and women are viewed as equals and where connectedness, nurturance, sharing, and humility are valued as highly as ambition, status, and power over others.

In this tradition, Adrienne Rich (1976) discusses what mothers might wish to instill in their sons:

> What do we want for our sons? Women who have begun to challenge the values of patriarchy are haunted by this question. We want them to remain, in the deepest sense, sons of the mother, yet also to grow into themselves, to discover new ways of being men even as we are discovering new ways of being women. We could wish that there were more fathers—not one, but many—to whom

they could also be sons, fathers with the sensitivity and
commitment to help them into a manhood in which they would
not perceive women as the sole sources of nourishment and solace.
(p. 210)

A new twist has been added to the envisioning process by feminists
who have uncovered early, nonpatriarchal societies and have been
asking the question why, if gender equality was once the rule, it cannot
be again. Maria Gimbutas (1974, 1989), Riane Eisler (1987), Elinor
Gadon (1989), and others point out that certain neolithic cultures—in
Turkey, Eastern Europe, and the Near East (Crete's culture is one of the
last survivors)—were based on pervasive gender equality, and natural
cycles were an important part of cultural life. Women were venerated
and served as priestesses in religious rites. Archeological evidence
suggests this veneration was based on women's role in procreation.
Eisler insists women did not rule—that would merely be a reversal of
patriarchal rule while retaining its basic form—rather they were given
equal place in society and their contributions were honored. Interestingly, archeologists have also discovered that these neolithic societies
had relatively advanced technology for their time—indoor plumbing,
for instance—and that there was much less class stratification than
there is in modern societies. According to these feminists, even if
patriarchal hunting and warrior peoples conquered and laid waste to the
agrarian societies that venerated women and their natural cycles, what
once was might be again.

The question has been raised in academic circles whether Gimbutas' evidence is too preliminary and sketchy to support the sweeping
generalizations she makes (Barnett, 1992). Clearly, as soon as we begin
to speculate on the basis of archeological evidence about the details of
everyday life in an age prior to recorded history we are merely projecting
our modern assumptions backward through time. Feminist theories
about neolithic Goddess/ Priestess cultures have this built-in bias and,
as history, are necessarily tentative. But this is not the main point.
These feminists, in their speculations about the distant past, are saying
something important about what is today and what might be in the
future. Their speculations, like Freud's about the "primal horde," serve
merely as metaphor. Like Ruth Benedict (1934), Margaret Mead
(1949), and other "cultural relativists" in anthropology, these feminists
are debunking the notion that gender roles are innate, universal, and
unchanging. They are providing a speculative interpretation of the
distant past so that we can envision a very different future.

Contrast the work of Gimbutas, Eisler, and other feminists with
the tendency among some men to idealize a preindustrial past when

drumming, rituals, and mentorship provided a conduit for the male quest. There is a dramatic difference between these men's and women's references to the distant past. For Gimbutas and Eisler, gender relations in our historical past provide hope for improvement, while men's nostalgia tends to focus instead on what they see as proof of their view of what it means to be a man.

Other men have different interpretations. Mark Gerzon (1982), for example, offers a study of heroes. Gerzon describes five traditional men's hero images: the frontiersman, the soldier, the expert, the breadwinner, and the man of God. Then he ponders the transition to a new kind of society where there will be different male heroes, including the healer, the companion, the mediator, and the nurturer. Gerzon interviews a man he feels fits the description of the hero as healer, Tom Mossmiller, a founder of the National Organization for Men Against Sexism (NOMAS) who was working at that time at a shelter for battered women and children, counseling the men who do the battering. Gerzon quotes Mossmiller:

> A lot of people think I work for a feminist counseling center only because I want to protect women. And I do. I do not want them to get beaten up. But I also work with abusive men because I care about them. They may not have any scars showing, but inside they're just as torn up as the women they hurt. I want to help them get in touch with the gentle, caring, sensitive person inside them. They do not like the kind of men they have become. My commitment is to help them change. (p. 241)

What if men were to look forward to a world where competition and domination no longer reign, where men as well as women strive to stay in touch with "the gentle, caring, sensitive person inside them?" Would men who, according to traditional definitions of the gender norm, fit in now, fit in then? Would PMS still be viewed as a category of mental disorder or would men more likely question their obsessive quest for steadiness? Would the men's movement stigmatize softness and homosexuality in men, or would there be a concerted effort to transcend homophobia, sexual compulsivity, and an obsession with pornography? Who would be viewed as the oddball, the man who values personal relationships and childrearing responsibilities or the one who ignores family life in order to concentrate on excelling at work and climbing higher in the hierarchy? How would we define power? These are the kinds of questions we must ask if we are to succeed, collectively, at redrawing the lines that presently constrict men's lives.

CHAPTER ELEVEN

Conclusion: Redefining Power

Men tend to define power very narrowly as the power to impose one's will over others. In order to enhance his power a man must very early in life begin achieving respect, a reputation, a position of authority, good connections, status, wealth, and the like. And this is connected to our notion of manliness. As long as men believe that they must be concerned above all else with their place in a hierarchy, and that the only choices they have are an ambitious climb to the top or a fall to the bottom of the heap, we will continue to maintain a steady pace, fear dependency, feel isolated from others, compensate for our inadequacies by oppressing women and gays, and continue to be uncertain about our adequacy no matter what heights we attain.

Kenneth Boulding (1990) distinguishes three dimensions of power. *Threat power* is the kind that permits one to get one's way in the face of challenges from others. This is that narrow sense of power, the ability to force opponents to give in for fear of unpleasant consequences. Then there is *exchange power*, the ability to produce and exchange objects of value. And the third is *integrative power*, the ability to achieve what one desires through love, nurturing, loyalty, and other positive forms of connection with people. It is only because men feel that they lack integrative power that they rely so one-sidedly on threat power, for instance beating their wives when they feel unable to attain by any other means the degree of unconditional love and respect they crave.

Steve Smith (1991) applies Boulding's three dimensions of power to the study of masculinity, pointing out that in our society the uses of power are organized along gender lines, men relying more on *threat power* while women rely more on *integrative power*. According to Smith:

> If power is exclusively threat power, men are indeed the more powerful sex. But if power includes the ability to bring about any perceived good—including meeting one's own basic needs—then integrative power becomes central to the analysis of power differentials between the sexes. Itself responsible for many of the greatest of human goods, integrative power is frequently exercised more effectively by women. Many men are sadly deficient in integrative power precisely because they have assumed a greater role in the exercise of threat power. They thus become dependent upon women to meet basic human needs, while (in the service of threat power) denying their very dependency. Once we have overthrown the illusion of threat power as all-encompassing, the costs to men are glaringly evident. (p. 25)

There are two aspects of power that warrant redefinition. One involves goals and values, the other involves the actual wielding of power. In terms of goals and values, men traditionally define power in relation to their sense of themselves as "real men." What makes one feel more like a "real man" is what one calls power. Even men who involve themselves fully in the rearing of children or the caring for people who are dying of AIDS sometimes feel they are less a man for it. It is as if a part of these men still buys into the American dream and thinks the most powerful men are the ones who earn huge salaries and sit among the power elite. Then they compare and decide they are relatively less powerful, less successful, and therefore less of a man. If things are to change for the better, we must redefine power so that we can feel powerful while doing tasks that are not traditional for men. Of course, this means men must assign more value to *integrative power* and less to *threat power* and *exchange power*.

An incident from a men's therapy group I conduct illustrates the point. Two group members who regularly spar with each other at meetings begin a dialogue about what it is about the other that rubs each the wrong way. What part of each man is set off by the antics of the other, and what earlier relationship(s) with a man make this combative relationship seem so familiar to each? Both explore earlier relationships with fathers, brothers, and teachers that come to mind. Both say they feel intimidated by the other and find it difficult to open up and be vulnerable in the other's presence. The group confronts the two, demanding to know why they have to be so combative all the time. The group wants this duo to resolve their differences so there can be more trust and openness at meetings.

A few weeks later one of the two men confesses to the group he is feeling very depressed, wonders whether it is worth going on, and has no clue as to the cause of his depression. This degree of vulnerability is quite uncharacteristic for him. The man with whom he usually spars is silent during that session, but at the next weekly meeting says he was quite moved by the other's confession that he did not know the cause of his depression. The group discusses the tendency among men to act intimidating just when they feel vulnerable. At this point a third member asks the man who was depressed whether he really achieves what he wants by being combative. He responds: "Not really. It feels better to be close to you guys, even while I'm feeling miserable, and to be in this conversation right now." In other words; if the goal is to be able to lord it over other men as one does in a business rivalry or legal battle, intimidation and male posturing work; but if the goal is to end one's sense of isolation and feel connected to others, vulnerability and trust make one more effective and powerful.

As a society, should the first priority be the maximization of short-term profit or should it be the creation of a just society in which everyone has a job and a roof over their heads? Should we continue to sink a huge proportion of our tax dollar into the race for global military dominance, or should we shift resources into alternative uses of advanced technology, for instance, figuring out ways to feed everyone and still preserve a livable environment? Would we be less powerful as a nation if we were to put more of our resources into figuring out ways to make the largest number of people in our society happy, but in the process we accumulated less financial and military *threat power* in the international arena? In fact, because the world has changed it is no longer reasonable to expect the United States to dominate the globe economically as it did in the post-World War II era—unless, that is, we attempt to continue our domination by military means, a disastrous course. But if we are to convert our social priorities and embark on a peaceful path of international collaboration, we will have to reconstruct our notion of masculinity, of what it means to be a "real man." We will have to redefine power in a way that permits men to feel powerful while they rear children, care for the ill, develop better quality intimacies, and so forth.

I mentioned that there are two aspects of power that warrant redefining. The second involves the wielding of power. If the men who value their *integrative power* end up giving away their power in the public arena, then control of this society will remain in the hands of the one-dimensional wielders of *threat power* who have succeeded in practically destroying the environment and bringing us to the brink of world war. If men who would change all this redefine power and reorder their priorities, will not that make them, as a group, less powerful in society? Because this has never happened in a modern society, we cannot know the answer. But we can attempt, collectively, to make that answer a resounding no. Men who utilize their *integrative power* as much as their *threat power* can be just as powerful, or more powerful, as those who currently wield power. This must be the case if things are to change for the better.

I believe that men who utilize their *integrative power* can be more powerful as a social force than they would be if they, like traditional men, relied almost exclusively on their *threat power*. Again, the lesson comes from the women's movement. Women were able to improve their situation, their solidarity with other women, and the quality of their lives by refusing to join men in a battle involving *threat power* alone. They insisted the personal was political, and taught us it could be. And in the process they demonstrated how powerful their *integrative power* could make them. For instance, women's friendships and capacity to meet in groups and talk about deeply personal issues make them very effective as organizers for social change. If there is any doubt, consider the way the women's movement has thrown the spotlight on sexual harassment at work, and the greater leverage women now have to put a halt to it. Men must learn that connectedness with others can boost one's power, and that by working together we can be even more powerful, especially if we figure out ways to collaborate without constructing new hierarchies and rivalries.

A large number of men are discovering a new kind of power, the kind that is expressed in having a wonderful circle of intimates and feeling secure because of it, the power that derives from knowing one is living according to one's principles even if that means one does not accumulate all one might, the kind that comes from sharing the burden with others one can respect as equals. In a community of equals a new kind of power can be realized, not the kind where a man stands alone and conquers real and imagined enemies; rather, a man would be able to discuss problems with a network of sympathetic people who might help him devise a collaborative strategy for solving a large array of problems and coping with a variety of threats. When I see men at gatherings celebrating their newfound sense of brotherhood and the relief they feel that they are not as totally alone in the universe as they once felt they were, I know I am part of something that is very powerful and I feel powerful being a part.

Once men begin to expand upon what Boulding terms their *integrative power*, a whole set of connections become obvious. Men who are attuned to the plight of others are not able to ignore sexual harassment at work, homelessness, racism, drastic cutbacks in social welfare programs, inattention to the plight of AIDS sufferers, ecological disasters such as the destruction of the rain forests and the ozone layer, and the threat of war and nuclear annihilation.

Men who get in touch with their feminine side, and begin to value their role as father, friend, and team player, need not give away their power in the public arena. In fact, by working collaboratively with others who share a vision of better gender relations, men will discover a whole new level of power. And, by their example, they will begin to redefine masculinity as well as power.

Vying for power in the public arena involves a large organizational effort. Massive public involvement is needed to win abortion rights, effective affirmative action, decent jobs for men and women, affordable childcare, and so on. I am not ready to propose a specific political program, that will require discussion among a large number of people. But I am saying we need to become more active in social struggles if we are to change anything. Many men's groups as well as individual men have joined women's struggles to "take back the night"; end domestic violence, date rape, and child abuse; and many straights have joined gays in the struggle against AIDS. Men's groups and organizations could also join their blue collar brothers and sisters on picket lines protesting plant closures and joblessness. And men could join their brothers among the minorities in protesting the dismantling of inner city schools, the unavailability of affordable housing and rewarding work opportunities, and the inattention to people of color who are dying of AIDS as well as other diseases.

Changing gender relations is not merely a matter of social struggles. Personal relationships must change as well. As a large number of people engage in collaborative childrearing, our definitions of manliness and power change. Men who work with men who batter are redefining power in the domestic realm, teaching men who feel inadequate that they can feel more powerful on account of caring relationships with women and children (*integrative power*) than they ever would on account of their ability to beat and abuse them (*threat power*, see Sonkin & Durphy, 1982; Kivel, 1992). Black men who go to inner city schools to talk with youths about sex, drugs, and alternatives to enlistment in the military are redefining power for these youngsters, teaching them that a quick buck and the ability to lord it over others is not the only way to feel powerful. There are many other examples of the new kinds of heroes we already have among us.

I began this book with a discussion of men who abhor domination from an early age and support women's struggles for equality, even while they are unable to stand up to the women in their lives and do not accomplish all they might at work for fear of becoming brutes.

These men must find ways to stand up for their own rights—in personal relationships, at work, and in the public arena—or else men who have no qualms about the suffering of others will continue to wield most of the power in this society. To the extent men lack a vision of a better society in which one does not have to be a brute to have a voice in the halls of power—a vision that provides a third alternative to the either/or dichotomy of winners and losers in the (*threat*) power game—they settle for lives that are less than fully vital. The challenge that confronts men is to find ways to be powerful without oppressing anyone, and in the process to redefine power, heroism, and masculinity. This is an immense challenge. And men will never meet it in isolation. We need new kinds of bonds among men and between men and women, straight and gay, if we are to construct, collectively, new forms of masculinity and new and better gender relations.

References

Abbott, F. (1990). The Image and the Act: Men, Sex and Love. In *Men & Intimacy*, ed. F. Abbott. Freedom, CA: Crossing Press, 231–239.

Adler, A. (1912). Psychical Hermaphrodism and the Masculine Protest—The Cardinal Problem of Nervous Diseases. In *Individual Psychology*, trans. P. Radin. London: Routledge & Kegan Paul, 1950, 16–22.

Adler, A. (1927). *Understanding Human Nature*. New York: Greenberg. Excerpt reprinted in *Psychoanalysis and Women*, ed. J. B. Miller. New York: Penguin, 1973, 40–50.

Alcoholics Anonymous. (1939). *The Big Book*. New York: A.A. World Services, Inc.

Allen, H. (1984). At the Mercy of Her Hormones: Premenstrual Tension and the Law. *m/f*, 9, 19–44.

American Psychiatric Association. (1987). Diagnostic and Statistical Manual of Mental Disorders. Third Edition, Revised. Washington, DC: Author.

Astrachan, A. (1986). *How Men Feel: Their Response to Women's Demands for Equality and Power*. New York: Doubleday.

Barnett, W. (1992). Review of Maria Gimbutas, *The Language of the Goddess* (1989). *American Journal of Archaeology*, 96(1), 170–171.

Barz, H. (1991). *For Men, Too: A Grateful Critique of Feminism*. Wilmette, Il: Chiron Publications.

Basaglia, F. (1980). Breaking the Circuit of Control. In *Critical Psychiatry*, ed. D. Ingleby. New York: Pantheon, 184–192.

Bayer, R. (1981). *Homosexuality and American Psychiatry*. New York: Basic Books.

Beane, J. (1990). Choiceful Sex, Intimacy and Relationships for Gay and Bisexual Men. In *Men & Intimacy*, ed. F. Abbott. Freedom, CA: Crossing Press, 157–165.

Bellah, R., Madsen, R., Sullivan, W., Swidler, A., and Tipton, S. (1985). *Habits of the Heart: Individualism and Commitment in American Life*. Berkeley: University of California Press.

Benedict, R. (1934). *Patterns of Culture*. Boston: Houghton Mifflin.

Benjamin, J. (1988). *The Bonds of Love: Psychoanalysis, Feminism and the Problem of Domination*. New York: Pantheon Books.

Bergman, S. J. (1991). Men's Psychological Development: A Relational Perspective. Wellesley, MA: The Stone Center Work in Progress No. 33.

Bernardez, T. (1982). The Female Therapist in Relation to Male Roles. In *Men in Transition: Theory and Therapy*, eds. K. Solomon and N. B. Levy. New York: Plenum Press, 439–462.

Bernstein, A. (1989). *Yours, Mine, and Ours: How Families Change When Remarried Parents Have a Child Together*. New York: Charles Scribner's Sons.

Bettelheim, B. (1971). Obsolete Youth: Toward a Psychograph of Adolescent Rebellion. In *Adolescent Psychiatry, Vol. 1*, eds. S. Feinstein, P. Giovacchini, and A. Miller. New York: Jason Aronson, 14–39.

Biller, H.B. (1970). Father Absence and the Personality Development of the Male Child. *Developmental Psychology*, 2(2), 181–201.

Blauner, R. (1991). The Men's Movement and its Analysis of the Male Malaise. Unpublished manuscript.

Bliss, S. (1990). Interview by Milt Schwartz. *Sober Times*, 5(9), 22–24.

Blos, P. (1984). Son and Father. *Journal of the American Psychoanalytic Association*, 32, 301–324.

Bly, R. (1982). What Men Really Want. Interview with Keith Thompson. *New Age*, May, 30–51.

Bly, R. (1989). The Male Mode of Feeling. Audiotape. Pacific Grove, CA: Oral Tradition Archives.

Bly, R. (1990). *Iron John: A Book About Men*. New York: Addison-Wesley.

Boehm, R. (1932). The Femininity Complex in Men. *International Journal of Psychoanalysis*, 11, 444–469.

Bograd, M. (1990). Women Treating Men. *The Family Therapy Networker*, May/June, 54–60.

Boulding, K. E. (1990). *Three Faces of Power*. Newbury Park, CA: Sage.

Brittan, A. (1989). *Masculinity and Power*. New York: Basil Blackwell.

Brod, H., Ed. (1987). *The Making of Masculinities: The New Men's Studies*. Boston: Allen & Unwin.

Brod, H. (1988). Pornography and the Alienation of Male Sexuality. *Social Theory and Practice*, 14(3), 265–284.

Cabaj, R.P. (1985). Homophobia: A Hidden Factor in Psychotherapy. *Contemporary Psychiatry*, 4(3), 135–137.

Cahill, T. (1990). Prison Rape: Torture in the American Gulag. In *Men & Intimacy*, ed. F. Abbott. Freedom, CA: Crossing Press, 31–36.

Caldicott, H. (1984). *Missile Envy: The Arms Race and Nuclear War*. New York: Bantam.

Carpenter, E. (1916). Selected Insights. In *Gay Spirit: Myth and Meaning*, ed. M. Thompson. New York: St. Martin's Press, 1987, 152–164.

Carrigan, T., Connell, B., and Lee, J. (1987). Toward a New Sociology of Masculinity. In *The Making of Masculinities: The New Men's Studies*, ed. H. Brod. Boston: Allen & Unwin, 63–100.

Carvalho, R. R. N. (1982). Paternal Deprivation in Relation to Narcissistic Damage. *Journal of Analytical Psychology, 27*, 341–356.

Cash, W. J. (1941). *Mind of the South*. New York: Alfred A. Knopf.

Cathie, S. (1987). What Does it Mean to Be a Man? *Free Associations, 8,* 7–33.

Chesler, P. (1976). *Women and Madness*. New York: Avon.

Chodorow, N. (1978). *The Reproduction of Mothering: Psychoanalysis and the Sociology of Gender*. Berkeley: University of California Press.

Coleman, J. (1973). Surviving Psychotherapy. In *Radical Psychology*, ed. P. Brown, New York: Harper Colophon, 497–508.

Connell, R. (1987). *Gender and Power: Society, the Person and Sexual Politics*. Stanford: Stanford University Press.

Connell, R. (1989). Cool Guys, Swots and Wimps: The Interplay of Masculinity and Education. *Oxford Review of Education, 15*(3), 291–303.

Connell, R. (1990). A Whole New World: Remaking Masculinity in the Context of the Environmental Movement. *Gender and Society, 4*(4), 452–478.

Connell, R. (1992). Drumming Up the Wrong Tree. *Tikkun, 7*(1), 31–36.

Dinnerstein, D. (1976). *The Mermaid and the Minotaur*. New York: Harper & Row.

Dreiser, T. (1900, 1959). *Sister Carrie*. Boston: Houghton Mifflin.

Duroche, L. L. (1991). Men Fearing Men: On the Nineteenth-Century Origins of Modern Homophobia. *Men's Studies Review, 8*(3), 3–7.

Dworkin, A. (1989). *Pornography: Men Possessing Women*. New York: E.P. Dutton.

Ehrenreich, B. (1983). *The Hearts of Men: American Dreams and the Flight from Commitment*. New York: Anchor.

Ehrensaft, D. (1987). *Parenting Together*. New York: Free Press.

Ehrensaft, D. (1990). Feminists Fight (for) Fathers. *Socialist Review, 90*(4), 57–80.

Eisler, R. (1987). *The Chalice & the Blade: Our History, Our Future*. New York: Harper & Row.

Ellis, K. (1990). I'm Black and Blue from the Rolling Stones and I'm Not Sure How I Feel about It: Pornography and the Feminist Imagination. In *Women, Class and the Feminist Imagination: A Socialist-Feminist Reader*, eds. K. Hansen and I. Philipson. Philadelphia: Temple University Press, 431–450.

Erkel, R. T. (1990). The Birth of a Movement. *Family Therapy Networker*, May/June, 26–35.

Faludi, S. (1991). *Backlash: The Undeclared War on American Women*. New York: Crown.

Fanon, F. (1965). *Studies in a Dying Colonialism*. New York: Monthly Review Press.

Feuer, L. (1969). *The Conflict of Generations: The Character and Significance of Student Movements*. New York: Basic Books.

Fine, R. (1988). *Troubled Men: The Psychology, Emotional Conflicts, and*

Forstein, M. (1988). Homophobia: an Overview. *Psychiatric Annals, 18*(1), 33–36.

Frank, B. (1987). Hegemonic Heterosexual Masculinity. *Studies in Political Economy, 24,* 159–170.

Franklin, C. (1987). Surviving the Institutional Decimation of Black Males: Causes, Consequences and Intervention. In *The Making of Masculinities*, ed. H. Brod. Boston: Allen & Unwin, 155–170.

Freud, S. (1913a). Totem and Taboo. *Standard Edition, 13,* 1–164. London: Hogarth, 1957–1961.

Freud, S. (1913b). Further Recommendations on the Technique of Psychoanalysis: On Beginning the Treatment. *Standard Edition, 12,* 121–44. London: Hogarth, 1957–1961.

Freud, S. (1921). Group Psychology and the Analysis of the Ego. *Standard Edition, 18,* 67–145. London: Hogarth, 1957–1961.

Freud, S. (1925). Some Psychical Consequences of the Anatomical Distinctions Between the Sexes. *Standard Edition, 19,* 248–260. London: Hogarth, 1957–1961.

Freud, S. (1937). Analysis Terminable and Interminable. *Standard Edition, 23,* 209–254. London: Hogarth, 1957–1961.

Friedman, R. (1986). The Psychoanalytic Model of Male Homosexuality: A Historical and Theoretical Critique. *The Psychoanalytic Review, 73,* 483–519.

Fromm, E. (1941). *Escape From Freedom.* New York: Holt, Rinehart & Winston.

Fromm, E. (1962). *Beyond the Chains of Illusion.* New York: Trident Press.

Fromm, E. (1973). *The Anatomy of Human Destructiveness.* New York: Holt, Rinehart & Winston.

Gadon, E. W. (1989). *The Once & Future Goddess: A Symbol for Our Time.* San Francisco: Harper & Row.

Gay, P. (1988). *Freud: A Life for Our Time.* New York: W.W. Norton.

Genet, J. (1966). *Miracle of the Rose.* New York: Grove Press.

Gerzon, M. (1982). *A Choice of Heroes: The Changing Face of American Manhood.* Boston: Houghton Mifflin.

Gilligan, C. (1982). *In a Different Voice: Psychological Theory and Women's Development.* Cambridge: Harvard University Press.

Gimbutas, M. (1974). *The Goddesses and Gods of Old Europe: Myths and Cult Images.* Berkeley: University of California Press.

Gimbutas, M. (1989). *The Language of the Goddess.* San Francisco: Harper San Francisco.

Goffman, E. (1961). *Asylums: Essays on the Social Situation of Mental Patients and Other Inmates.* Chicago: Aldine.

Goldberg, A. (1973). Psychotherapy of Narcissistic Injury. *Archives of General Psychiatry, 28,* 722–726.

Gordon, B., and Meth, R. (1990). Men as Husbands. In *Men in Therapy: The Challenge of Change,* eds. R. L. Meth and R. S. Pasick. New York: Guilford Press, 54–87.

Gordon, B. and Pasick, R. S. (1990). Changing the Nature of Friendships between Men. In *Men in Therapy: The Challenge of Change*, eds. R. L. Meth and R. S. Pasick. New York: Guilford Press, 261–278.

Greenson, R. (1968). Dis-identifying from mother. *International Journal of Psychoanalysis, 49,* 370–374.

Griffin, S. (1981). *Pornography and Silence: Culture's Revenge Against Nature.* New York: Harper & Row.

Hammond, D., and Jablow, A. (1987). Gilgamesh and the Sundance Kid: The Myth of Male Friendship. In *The Making of Masculinities: The New Men's Studies,* ed. H. Brod. Boston: Allen & Unwin, 241–258.

Havel, V. (1990). On Kafka. *New York Review of Books,* September 27.

Henry, J. (1963). *Culture Against Man.* New York: Random House.

Hillman, J. (1964). Betrayal. The Guild of Pastoral Psychology, Guild Lecture No. 128.

Hillman, J. (1990). Interview by Michael Ventura. *L A Weekly (June 1–7),* 12, 26.

Hochschild, A. (1989). *The Second Shift: Inside the Two-Job Marriage.* New York: Viking.

Horney, K. (1924). On the Genesis of the Castration Complex in Women. *International Journal of Psychoanalysis, 4,* 50–65.

Horney, K. (1926). The Flight from Womanhood: The Masculinity Complex in Women as Viewed by Men and by Women. *International Journal of Psychoanalysis, 7,* 324–339.

Horney, K. (1935). The Problem of Feminine Masochism. *Psychoanalytic Review, 12,*(3), 241–257.

Jay, M. (1973). *The Dialectical Imagination: A History of the Frankfurt School and the Institute of Social Research, 1923–1950.* Boston: Little, Brown.

Jones, E. (1927). Early Development of Female Sexuality. *International Journal of Psychoanalysis, 8,* 459–472.

Jordan, J. (1989). Relational Development: Therapeutic Implications of Empathy and Shame. Wellesley, MA: The Stone Center Work in Progress No. 39.

Jordan, J, Kaplan, A., Miller, J.B., Stiver, I.P., and Surrey, J. L. (1991). *Women's Growth in Connection: Writings from the Stone Center.* New York: Guilford Press.

Keen, S. (1991). *Fire in the Belly: On Being a Man.* New York: Bantam Books.

Kernberg, O. (1975). *Borderline Conditions and Pathological Narcissism.* New York: Jason Aronson.

Kessler, L. (1983). *Orphans.* New York: Grove Press.

Kessler, S. J., and McKenna, W. (1978). *Gender: An Ethnomethodological Approach.* New York: Wiley.

Kimmel, M. (1987). The Contemporary "Crisis" of Masculinity in Historical Perspective. In *The Making of Masculinities: The New Men's Studies,* ed. H. Brod. Boston: Allen & Unwin, 121–154.

Kimmel, M., ed. (1990). *Men Confront Pornography.* New York: Crown.

Kimmel, M. (1991). Issues for Men in the 1990s. *Changing Men, 22,* 4–17.

Kivel, P. (1992). *Men's Work: How to Stop the Violence That Tears Our Lives Apart.* Center City, MN: Hazeldon.

Kohut, H. (1971). *The Analysis of the Self: A Systematic Approach to the Psychoanalytic Treatment of Narcissistic Personality Disorders.* New York: International Universities Press.

Kovel, J. (1981). *The Age of Desire: Case Histories of a Radical Psychoanalyst.* New York: Pantheon.

Kovel, J. (1990). The Antidialectic of Pornography. In *Men Confront Pornography,* ed. M. Kimmel. New York: Crown, 153–167.

Kroeber, A. L. (1920). Totem and Taboo: An Ethnologic Psychoanalysis. *American Anthropologist, 22,* 48–55.

Kroeber, A. L. (1939). Totem and Taboo in Retrospect. *American Journal of Sociology, 45*(3), 446–451.

Kundera, M. *The Book of Laughter and Forgetting.* New York: Alfred A. Knopf.

Kupers, T. (1986). The Dual Potential of Brief Psychotherapy. *Free Association, 6,* 80–99.

Kupers, T. (1988). *Ending Therapy: The Meaning of Termination.* New York: New York University Press.

Kupers, T. (1990). Feminist Men, *Tikkun, 5*(4), 35–38.

Kupers, T. (1993). Psychotherapy and the Role of Activism. *Community Mental Health Journal,* in press.

Laing, R. D. (1967). *The Politics of Experience.* New York: Ballantine.

Laing, R. D. (1969). *The Politics of the Family.* Toronto: CBC Publications.

Laphan, J., Producer. (1990). *Changing Roles, Changing Lives,* a film. Boston: Oasis Films.

Lasch, C. (1979). *The Culture of Narcissism: American Life in an Age of Diminishing Expectations.* New York: Norton & Co.

Lerner, M. (1991). *Surplus Powerlessness: The Psychodynamics of Everyday Life and the Psychology of Individual and Social Transformation.* New York: Humanities Press.

Levine, S. (1992). Exploration and Healing, a Workshop. Oakland, California, January 18.

Levinson, D. (1978). *The Seasons of a Man's Life.* New York: Ballantine.

Lidz, T., and Lidz, R. (1986). Turning Women Things into Men: Masculinization in Papua New Guinea. *The Psychoanalytic Review, 73*(4), 553–566.

Lodge, D. (1978). *Changing Places.* London: Penguin.

Loewald, H. (1980). On the Therapeutic Action of Psychoanalysis. In *Papers on Psychoanalysis.* New Haven: Yale University Press, 221–256.

Lopate, P. (1990). Renewing Sodom and Gomorrah. In *Men Confront Pornography,* ed. M. Kimmel. New York: Crown, 25–33.

Maccoby, M. (1976). *The Gamesmen: The New Corporate Leaders.* New York: Simon & Schuster.

Malyon, A. (1982). Psychotherapeutic Implications of Internalized Homophobia in Gay Men. In *Homosexuality and Psychotherapy,* ed. J. Gonsiorek. New York: The Haworth Press.

Marcus, E. (1988). *The Male Couple's Guide to Living Together*. New York: Harper & Row.

Marcuse, H. (1955). *Eros and Civilization*. Boston: Beacon.

Marcuse, H. (1978). *The Aesthetic Dimension: Toward a Critique of Marxist Aesthetics*. Boston: Beacon Press.

Markowitz, L. (1991). Homosexuality: Are We Still in the Dark? *Family Therapy Networker*, Jan/Feb, 27–35.

Marmor, J. (1980). Homosexuality and the Issue of Mental Illness. In *Homosexual Behavior: a Modern Reappraisal*, ed. J. Marmor. New York: Basic Books.

McGill, M.E. (1985). The McGill Report on Male Intimacy. New York: Holt, Reinhart.

Mead, M. (1949). *Male and Female: A Study of the Sexes in a Changing World*. New York: William Morrow.

Meissner, W.M. (1978). Conceptualization of Marriage and Family Dynamics from a Psychoanalytic Perspective. In *Marriage and Marital Therapy*, eds. T.J. Paolino and B.S. McCrady. New York: Brunner/Mazel, 25–88.

Men Against Pornography. (1990). Is Pornography Jerking You Around? In *Men Confront Pornography*, ed. M. Kimmel. New York: Crown, 293–296.

Meth, R. (1990). The Road to Masculinity. In *Men in Therapy: The Challenge to Change*, eds. R. Meth and R. L. Pasick. New York: Guilford Press, 3–34.

Meyers, H. (1986). How do Women Treat Men? In *The Psychology of Men: New Psychoanalytic Perspectives*, eds. G. Fogel, F. Lane and R. Liebert. New York: Basic Books, 262–276.

Michaelis, D. (1983). *The Best of Friends: Profiles of Extraordinary Friendships*. New York: Morrow.

Miller, A. (1981). *Prisoners of Childhood: The Drama of the Gifted Child and the Search for the True Self*. New York: Basic Books.

Miller, J. B., ed. (1973). *Psychoanalysis and Women*. New York: Penguin Books.

Miller, J. B. (1976). *Toward a New Psychology of Women*. Boston: Beacon Press.

Miller, J. B. (1988). Connections, Disconnections and Violations. Wellesley, MA: Stone Center Work in Progress No. 33.

Miller, S. (1983). *Men and Friendship*. Bath, England: Gateway Books.

Mitchell, J. (1974). *Psychoanalysis and Feminism*. New York: Pantheon.

Mittscherlich, A. (1969). *Society Without the Father: A Contribution to Social Psychology*. New York: Harcourt, Brace & World.

Montagu, A. (1968). *Man and Aggression*. New York: Oxford University Press.

Moore, R., and Gillette, D. (1990). *King Warrior Magician Lover: Rediscovering the Archetypes of the Mature Masculine*. San Francisco: Harper San Francisco.

Morgan, R. (1980). Theory and Practice: Pornography and Rape. In *Take Back the Night: Women on Pornography*, ed. L. Lederer. New York: Morrow.

Morin, S., and Garfinkel, R. (1978a). Male Homophobia. *Journal of Social Issues*, 34(1), 29–47.

Morin, S., and Garfinkel, R. (1978b). Psychologists' attitudes Toward Homosexual Clients. *Journal of Social Issues*, 34(3), 101–112.

Mornell, P. (1979). *Passive Men, Wild Women*. New York: Ballantine.

Mumford, L. (1934). *Technics and Civilization*. New York: Harcourt, Brace and World.

Mura, D. (1987). A Male Grief: Notes on Pornography and Addiction. An Essay in the Thistle Series. Minneapolis: Milkweed Editions. Reprinted in *Men and Intimacy: Personal Accounts Exploring the Dilemmas of Modern Male Sexuality*, ed. F. Abbott. Freedom, CA: The Crossing Press, 1990, 66–76.

Murphy, T. (1984). Freud Reconsidered: Bisexuality, Homosexuality, and Moral Judgement. *Journal of Homosexuality*, 9, 65–77.

Murray, G. (1991). Homophobia in Robert Bly's *Iron John*. Paper presented at Sixteenth Annual Conference on Men and Masculinity, June, Tucson, Arizona.

O'Connor, T. (1990). A Day for Men. *Family Therapy Networker*, May/June, 36–39.

Olsen, P. (1981). *Sons and Mothers: Why Men Behave the Way They Do*. New York: Fawcett Crest.

Osherson, S. (1986). *Finding our Fathers: How a Man's Life is Shaped by His Relationship with His Father*. New York: Fawcett Columbine.

Osherson, S. (1992). *Wrestling with Love: How Men Struggle with Intimacy with Women, Children, Parents and Each Other*. New York: Fawcett.

Parsons, T., and Bales, R. F. (1955). *Family Socialization and Interaction Process*. Glencoe, IL: Free Press.

Pasick, R. L. (1990). Friendship Between Men. In *Men in Therapy: The Challenge of Change*, eds. R. Meth and R. L. Pasick. New York: Guilford Press, 108–130.

Pearce, D. (1978). The Feminization of Poverty: Women, Work and Welfare. *Urban and Social Change Review*, Feb, 28–37.

Perara, S. B. (1981). *Descent to the Goddess: A Way of Initiation for Women*. Toronto: Inner City Books.

Pharr, S. (1988). *Homophobia: A Weapon of Sexism*. Little Rock: Chardon Press.

Philipson, I. J. (1990). Beyond the Virgin and the Whore. In *Women, Class and the Feminist Imagination: A Socialist-Feminist Reader*, eds. K. Hansen and I. Philipson. Philadelphia: Temple University Press, 451–459.

Pleck, J. (1981). *The Myth of Masculinity*. Cambridge: The M.I.T. Press.

Radical Therapist Collective. (1971). *The Radical Therapist*. Producer, J. Agel. New York: Ballantine.

Redmountain, A. R. (1990). Men, Feminism and Pornography: An Attempt at Reconciliation. In *Men and Intimacy: Personal Accounts Exploring the Dilemmas of Modern Male Sexuality*, ed. F. Abbott. Freedom, CA: The Crossing Press, 77–80.

Reich, W. (1945). *The Sexual Revolution*. New York: Orgone Institute Press.

Reich, W. (1972). *Sex-Pol Essays: 1929–1934*, ed. L. Baxandall. New York: Random House.

Rich, A. (1976). *Of Woman Born: Motherhood as Experience and Institution*. New York: W.W. Norton.

Rilke, R. (1912). The Prodigal Son. In *Selected Poetry of Rainer Maria Rilke*, ed. S. Mitchell. New York: Vintage International, 1989, 109–115.

Ross, J. M. (1986). Beyond the Phallic Illusion: Notes on Man's Heterosexuality. In *The Psychology of Men: New Psychoanalytic Perspectives*, eds. G. Fogel, F. Lane, and R. Liebert. New York: Basic Books, 49–70.

Roth, P. (1991). *Patrimony*. New York: Simon & Schuster.

Rubin, G. (1981). Talking Sex: A conversation on Sexuality and Feminism. *Socialist Review*, 11(4), 43–62.

Rubin, L. (1983). *Intimate Strangers: Men and Women Together*. New York: Harper & Row.

Rubin, L. (1985). *Just Friends: The Role of Friendship in Our Lives*. New York: Harper & Row.

Sanday, P. R. (1990). *Fraternity Gang Rape: Sex, Brotherhood, and Privilege on Campus*. New York: New York University Press.

Scheff, T. (1966). *Being Mentally Ill*. Chicago: Aldine.

Schifellite, C. (1987). Beyond Tarzan and Jane Genes: Toward a Critique of Biological Determinism. In *Beyond Patriarchy: Essays by Men on Pleasure, Power, and Change*, ed. M. Kaufman. New York: Oxford University Press, 45–63.

Schwartz, F. (1989). Management Women and the New Facts of Life. *Harvard Business Review*, January.

Seidler, V. J. (1989). *Rediscovering Masculinity: Reason, Language and Sexuality*. New York: Routledge.

Seligman, E. (1982). The Half-Alive Ones. *Journal of Analytical Psychology*, 27, 1–20.

Sherrod, D. (1987). The Bonds of Men: Problems and Possibilities in Close Male Relationships. In *The Making of Masculinities: The New Men's Studies*, ed. H. Brod. Boston: Allen & Unwin, 213–241.

Shewey, D. (1992). Town Meetings in the Hearts of Men. *The Village Voice*, 37(6), 36–47.

Singer, I. B. (1962). The Strong Ones. In *In My Father's Court*. New York: Farrar, Strauss & Giroux, 219–224.

Smith, S. (1991). Men: Fear and Power. *Men's Studies Review*, 8(4), 20–27.

Soble, A. (1986). *Pornography: Marxism, Feminism and the Future of Sexuality*. New Haven: Yale University Press.

Solomon, K., and Levy, N., eds. (1982). *Men in Transition: Theory and Therapy*. New York: Plenum Press.

Sonkin, D. J., and Durphy, M. (1982). *Learning to Live Without Violence: A Handbook for Men*. Volcano, CA: Volcano Press.

Spitzer, R. L., Severino, S. K., Williams, J. B. and Parry, B.L. (1989). Late Luteal Phase Dysphoric Disorder and DSM-III-R. *American Journal of Psychiatry*, 146(7), 892–897.

Stacy, J. (1990). *Brave New Families: Stories of Domestic Upheaval in Late Twentieth Century America*. New York: Basic Books.

Stanton, D. (1991). Men Gone Mad: A Return to the Forest of the Mind. *Esquire*, 116(4), 113–124.

Sternbach, J. (1990). Opening Up. *The Family Therapy Networker*, May/June, 59–60.

Stoltenberg, J. (1989). *Refusing to be a Man: Essays on Sex and Justice*. New York: Meridian.

Tannen, D. (1991). *You Just Don't Understand: Women and Men in Conversation*. New York: Ballantine.

Thompson, C. (1942). Cultural Pressures in the Psychology of Women. *Psychiatry*, 5, 331–339.

Thompson, C. (1943). Penis Envy in Women. *Psychiatry*, 6, 123–125.

Thompson, E.P. (1967). Time, Work-discipline and Industrial Capitalism. *Past and Present*, 38, 56–97.

Thompson, M., ed. (1987). *Gay Spirit: Myth and Meaning*. New York: St. Martin's Press.

Tiger, L. (1969). *Men in Groups*. New York: Random House.

Warters, W. (1991). The Social Construction of Domestic Violence and the Implications of "Treatment" for Men Who Batter. *Men's Studies Review*, 8(2), 7–16.

Weeks, J. (1981) *Sex, Politics and Society: The Regulation of Sexuality Since 1800*. London: Longman.

Weinberg, M., and Bell, A. (1972). *Homosexuality: An Annotated Bibliography*. New York: Harper & Row.

Weir, L., and Casey, L. (1990) Subverting Power in Sexuality. In *Women, Class and the Feminist Imagination: A Socialist-Feminist Reader*, eds. K. Hansen and I. Philipson. Philadelphia: Temple University Press, 460–475.

Weisstein, N. (1970). "Kind, Kuche, Kirche" As Scientific Law: Psychology Constructs the Female. In *Sisterhood is Powerful*, ed. R. Morgan. New York: Vintage, 205–219.

Winnicott, D. W. (1971). *Playing and Reality*. New York: Basic Books.

Wolf, N. (1991). *The Beauty Myth: How Images of Beauty are Used Against Women*. New York: William Morrow & Company.

Woolf, V. (1929). *A Room of One's Own*. New York: Harcourt Brace Jovanovich.

Z, P. (1990). *A Skeptic's Guide to the Twelve Steps*. San Francisco: Hazelden/ Harper Collins.

Zilbergeld, B. (1990). Pornography as Therapy. In *Men Confront Pornography*, ed. M. Kimmel. New York: Crown, 120–122.

Zilboorg, G. (1944). Masculinity and femininity. *Psychiatry*, 7, 257–265.

Index